# A History of the Oral Surgery Club of Great Britain

**John Bradley**

Oxford, April 10.                                    PETER SHAW.

## Oral Surgery Club

Sir,—May I beg the courtesy of your columns to bring
to the notice of those of your readers who may be interested the fact that an oral surgery club has been formed
in England.

The club has been formed with the object of advancing
the science and art of oral surgery by providing for
contact between its members, also by arranging visits to
various British and foreign centres for the purpose of
seeing work done by different surgeons. Membership is
confined to those who specialize in oral surgery, or hold
a hospital or other appointment embracing surgery,
and who possess a medical or dental qualification. The
following have agreed to serve on the first committee:
*President :* Professor T. Talmage Read of Leeds;
*Members of the Committee :* Major S. H. Woods, A.D.C.,
Mr. T. Hall Felton of Grimsby. If any of your readers
are interested and would like information I would be
pleased to hear from them.—I am, etc.,

                                            R. S. Taylor,
88, Portland Place, W.1, April 8.          Honorary Secretary.

*Letter British Medical Journal.* April 17th 1937

ISBN 978-1501021220

July 2011

Updated 2014 & 2021

A History of the Oral Surgery Club
of Great Britain

*Cover: The first club meeting Leeds. 26th November 1937*

# Acknowledgements

The author wishes to thank members of the Club for some of the material used and for verbal contributions. The majority of the material was gained directly from the written archive, but acknowledgements are due to the Oxford University Press, the publishers of the Oxford Dictionary for the quotation of Wellington, and to Longmans, the publishers of the Chronicle of the 20th Century for the contemporary historical facts.

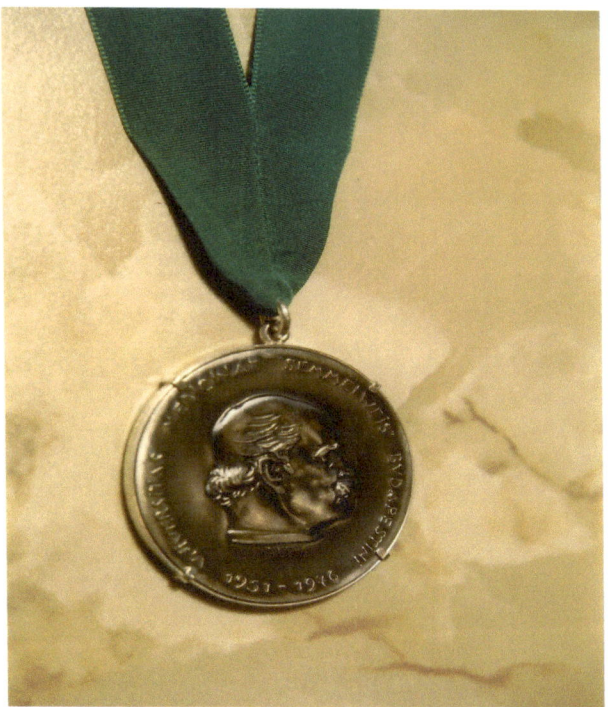

***The Semmelweis Medal.*** Presented to The Club in 1985 by the Semmelweis University of Medicine of Budapest. It has since has been worn as the Presidential medal.

# Contents

# The History of the Club

The Oral Surgery Club of Great Britain was the concept of one man, Rupert Sutton Taylor. He was probably the first person in the United Kingdom to restrict his practice to oral surgery and call himself an oral surgeon. Inevitably the character and nature of the Club reflect his personality to some extent. He was a great supporter of the general dental practitioner and was made an Honorary Fellow of the British Dental Association in 1969. Born an Irishman in County Wexford in 1905, he trained in dentistry at the Royal Dental Hospital and in medicine at the Middlesex Hospital, becoming a consultant at the Seamen's Hospital, Greenwich in 1930, at just twenty-five years old. He was appointed Clinical Assistant at the Westminster Hospital in 1929 and became consultant there in 1937. He was very much a military man, having joined the Territorial Army, RAMC in 1928 with a commission. He ran his clinical departments in good military style and when the Club was formed in 1937, he ran that along similar lines.

A confidential Army memo, which he enjoyed, ran "Rupert Sutton Taylor is a very able officer but inclined to be eccentric." This slight eccentricity still exists in the nature of the Club, and is mistaken by some as an anachronism. An example of his style of management within the Club occurred in 1965 on a visit to Lyons when a new member, a fellow countryman, was about to commit a misdemeanour which would have brought the Club disrespect. Taylor, who was Immediate Past President at the time, held a "Court Martial" in his hotel room and the miscreant was ordered back home, but he retained his membership.

In September 1936, when he was only thirty-one years old, he sent a letter to five people, Professor T. Talmage Read of Leeds, Professor Frank Wilkinson of Manchester, L. Wilson also of Manchester, T. Hall Fenton of Grimsby and Major S. H. Woods of the Millbank Military Hospital, London, proposing the formation of an oral surgery club and inviting them to form a steering committee. In that letter, his concept was to model the society on those existing at that time in medicine and surgery. Its object would be to advance the art and craft of oral surgery.

It was suggested that the society meet annually at a centre and pay visits to hospitals to study the work being carried out, and perhaps have a dinner. The response was enthusiastic, although L. Wilson's initial keenness seems to have faded rapidly as he never came into the picture. In the letters of reply, T. Hall Fenton wrote:

*that membership should be restricted to those who practise oral surgery to some extent and who are also willing to support the society actively.*

Active membership is a major criterion for continuing membership and demands attendance of at least one meeting in four. Members who do not meet this obligation, but with good reason, can be excused. Hall Fenton continues:

*In many Societies there are so many members who are willing to take whatever the Society offers but think that their obligation to put anything into it is completely discharged by the payment of a subscription.*

Attitudes do not seem to change, as this sentiment is often expressed today by those that are involved. He continues:

*…it should be a condition of membership that each member should be obliged to contribute annually to an aspect of the art of oral surgery: the papers might be printed and issued to members. Any member failing to contribute would automatically cease to be a member.*

What splendid stuff, and Hall Fenton was from Grimsby and not from some ivory tower. This admirable suggestion was not pursued for long but it gives a flavour that this society was to be active. Professor Wilkinson's letter was much shorter:

*Dear Taylor*

*I think your suggestion is a very good one. I would be prepared to join such a club, if formed.*

*It would, at any rate, give one an excuse for a good dinner.*

*With kind regards. Yours faithfully*

*F.C. Wilkinson*

Professor Talmage Read, in his reply to Taylor, really determined the nature of the Club. His reply of 15th September, 1936, is handwritten:

*My dear Taylor*

*Very many thanks for your letter. I think the idea of a surgical club is excellent and I would certainly support it. Have you considered those who would be eligible for membership as it does seem to be particularly specialised and might be more useful it if were kept exclusive. Have you any idea of the number who would be interested? I had a note from Mr Maloney regarding the meeting of the American Society – could you give me an idea of the nature of your paper and the scope? Am enclosing my last paper which you probably saw in the Journal.*

*With kindest regards.*

*Yours sincerely,*

*T. Talmage Read*

The implication was that you had to be established in oral surgical practice, and later we shall see that the number of members was to be limited to a relatively small number. This was quite different from the British Association of Oral Surgeons that was founded twenty-five years later where membership is inclusive, as any dentist or doctor with an interest in the subject can join.

The type of membership is echoed in Taylor's letter of 29th September 1936 and in the set of draft Rules he sent out with that letter.

*88 Portland Place, W1*

*Welbeck 6106*

*September 29th, 1936*

*Dear*

*I have had favourable replies regarding the proposed formation of an Oral Surgery Club from Mr T Hall Fenton of Grimsby, Professor T. Talmage Read of Leeds, Professor F.C. Wilkinson of Manchester, Mr L. Wilson of Manchester, and Major S. Ham Woods of Millbank. Including myself this makes a total of six, being all the people I have approached.*

*All these persons have some claim to be considered competent in Oral Surgery, and are either Specialists, or have charge of Hospital Departments devoted to the subject.*

*I enclose a draft of proposed provisional Rules, which I suggest should serve as a working constitution until such time as we can have an Inaugural Meeting.*

*I would very much like to have proposals as to the place and date of the first Meeting.*

*Yours sincerely, R.S. Taylor*

It is worth looking at the suggested constitution as it is of considerable interest and, seen in the context of the time, remarkable for its vision and insight. This had a considerable influence in the shaping of what is now the specialty of oral surgery.

*RULES*

*1. That the Club be known as the ORAL SURGERY CLUB.*

*2. That the object of the Club be to advance the Science and Art of Oral Surgery*

*3. That membership is confined to those persons who Specialize in Oral Surgery, or hold a Hospital or Public Appointment devoted to Oral Surgery.*

*4. That apart from the foundation Members all persons desirous of joining be required to produce evidence considered satisfactory by the Council that they are Specialists in Oral Surgery, or hold a Hospital or Public Appointment devoted to Oral Surgery.*

*5. That the affairs of the Club be managed by a Committee consisting of the President, the Secretary, and one other Member.*

*6. That the Subscription be £1.1.0 per year*

*7. That all cheques be signed by the Secretary and countersigned by the President*

*8. That all Members of the Club submit to the Committee once a year one original Paper, on some Subject relating to Oral Surgery of not less than 1000 words, or a description of a case they have treated of not less than 500 words. Such Paper or Case history to be suitably illustrated by Drawings, X Rays, Pathological Reports etc.*

*9. That these Rules be considered as provisional and shall only remain in force until such time as a permanent constitution is ratified by a General Meeting.*

It will be noted that firstly the original name was the Oral Surgery Club. The addition of "Great Britain" seems to have crept in during the immediate post-war years to indicate that an active membership was restricted to this country, but changes in the category of membership will be discussed later. Secondly, "the objects of the Club be to advance the science and art of oral surgery." The craft in surgical practice in 1936 was given greater emphasis then than it is today; indeed it is hardly mentioned, the emphasis now being on science.

Thirdly, membership was to be confined to those persons who specialise in oral surgery or hold a hospital or public appointment devoted to oral surgery. Following that, the credentials of those wishing to join needed to be scrutinised, and then the usual requirements for the smooth running of any organisation.

The eye alights on Hall Fenton's suggestion for Rule 8:

*That all Members of the Club submit to the Committee once a year one original Paper, on some Subject relating to Oral Surgery of not less than 1000 words, or a description of a case they have treated of not less than 500 words. Such Paper or Case history to be suitably illustrated by Drawings, X Rays, Pathological Reports etc.*

Continuing medical education in 1936 was regarded as a highly important activity; indeed the object of the Club was to pursue just that. It is sad that a small proportion of the profession in the late twentieth century seems to have forgotten this essential activity. The draft set of Rules seems to have been accepted without controversy. Wilkinson appears to be the only one commenting on them in writing:

*2nd October 1936*

*Dear Taylor*

*I think the rules submitted by you for the proposed club are adequate, at any rate for the time being.*

*As regards the meeting, I presume it will have to be in London and that we can borrow a suitable room from the British Dental Association or some other body of similar character.*

*On the whole I think that Friday evening or Saturday morning are most convenient times for me to get away.*

*Yours sincerely*

*F.C. Wilkinson*

The subject of the Rule Book usually generates seemingly endless debate, but here the objective of the Club was clearly foremost in their minds. However, it took them a little while to get together, but the date of Saturday 20th March 1937 was fixed, and the first meeting of the Steering Committee met at Sutton Taylor's house at 88 Portland Place, London, with Professor Talmage Read in the chair. Wilkinson and Wilson were unable to come, Wilkinson having written. The three remaining, other than Talmage Read, were of course, Taylor, Woods and Hall Fenton. Letters of support from the two absentees were read and the Oral Surgery Club was formally founded.

The Rules were then formulated along the lines proposed by Taylor the previous September. There are some further changes to the draft set: Rule 3, "...... or Public Appointment devoted to oral surgery" becomes

"…… or other Appointment embracing Oral Surgery, and who possess a Dental and/or Medical qualification." Rule 4 is simplified, Rule 5 allows the addition of another ordinary member to the Committee making two instead of one, and Rule 7 setting up the Bank Account.

*PROVISIONAL RULES*

*1. To be agreed to on the formation of the ORAL SURGERY CLUB.*

*2. That the Club be known as the ORAL SURGERY CLUB*

*3. That the objects of the Club be to advance the Science and Art of Oral - Surgery.*

*4. That Membership be confined to those persons who Specialize in Oral Surgery, or hold a Hospital or other Appointment embracing Oral Surgery and who possess a Dental and/or Medical qualification.*

*5. All persons desirous of joining be required to satisfy the Committee that they are eligible under Rule 4.*

*6. That the Club be administered by a Committee consisting of the President, the Secretary and two other Members.*

*7. That the Subscription be £1.1.0*

*8. That all Cheques be signed by the Secretary, Treasurer and counter signed by the President. All monies received on behalf of the Club be paid into the Club account at the Westminster Bank, 1 Cavendish Square, W.1.*

*9. That each Member of the Club shall submit on some Subject relating to Oral Surgery, or a description of a case he has treated. Such Paper or Case History to be suitably illustrated.*

*10. That these Rules be provisional and shall only remain in force until such time as a permanent constitution be ratified by a General Meeting.*

Hall Fenton's suggestion, embodied in Rule 9 to ensure continuing medical education, was modified in that the minimum length of submissions had been dropped.

Officers were then considered by the small group. Professor Talmage Read was elected President, Taylor was to be the Honorary Secretary and the Chairman proposed Woods and Hall Fenton be elected members of the Committee. At this point the first member of the Club to be invited was Professor Wilkinson, his name being proposed from the Chair. This was unanimously supported. L. Wilson was not proposed, which is a little curious – perhaps he withdrew, but there is no record of what actually happened.  There is another instance of an invitation to join being declined.

The meeting decided that the existence of the Club should be drawn to "the attention of the professional journals stating its objects" by a letter sent to six journals, including the British Dental Journal and the British Medical Journal.  Finally, the Steering Committee concluded that it would need to meet again; this time it did so on 19 June 1937 at Ye Olde Bell Hotel, Barnby Moor, Nottingham.  There were a number of important matters to be decided.

Firstly, the new members arising from the response to the advertisement in the professional journals had to be considered.  This was the only time when you could apply to join the Club; thereafter it has been by invitation only.  It is interesting to read the correspondence of the time.  Wilkinson was the first fully paid-up member.  He sent in his cheque for one guinea on 17 April 1937, possibly prompting Sutton Taylor to get out his own cheque book.  The first entries in the Cash Book show Wilkinson first and Taylor second, both recorded on the same date, 20 April 1937.

Wilkinson was very keen and had proposed Professor Humphreys of Birmingham before the inaugural meeting of 20 March 1937 in a letter to Taylor of 4 February 1937.  The letter of invitation of 12 February seems to have been unanswered.  Like L. Wilson, for some reason Professor Humphreys declined the invitation, which would have been very disappointing for Wilkinson.  The author met Professor Wilkinson on a number of occasions when he was well into his eighties, and even in old age he was sharp, keen and enthusiastic.  Taylor did well to recruit him.

However, all those who applied did not pass the scrutiny of the Committee at Barnby Moor, which obviously generated some debate as it is minuted:

> The President called the attention of the Committee to the fact that wine had been ordered for 7.30 and that it was now 7.45 the meeting adjourned for dinner.

They had only managed to complete the first two items on the agenda!  Brigadier Donald Taylor, a more junior officer then, wrote to apply, only to be turned down, probably because he was not senior enough.  Remember young Taylor was a consultant at a major teaching hospital by then, apart from being one at the Seamen's Hospital for the previous seven years  However, Donald Taylor was elected to the Club some nineteen years later in 1956.

The Committee finally proposed some sixteen names additional to Wilkinson to become the founder members of the Club (Appendix 1).

Having been revitalised by dinner, the meeting continued and they decided that the first General Meeting was to be at Leeds where Professor Talmage Read would arrange a scientific programme and "…. that the meeting should be devoted mainly to clinical subjects of interest to both dental and general surgeons." The Annual General Meetings of the club have retained this feature ever since. These meetings today recognise that the specialised field of oral and maxillofacial surgery does not exist in isolation from the rest of the surgical world and the "home" meetings mainly have lectures and papers from other disciplines both surgical and medical, with the occasional dental topic. These meetings are recognised for continuing medical education. The annual overseas meeting is devoted to the study of the specialty practised in that centre, and again are recognised for educational purposes.

Looking again at the list of founder members, there was a wide geographical spread and again this has been a feature of the club (Appendix 1). At one time, which cannot be dated but it was probably in the 1950s, the percentage coming from London was restricted to twenty-five per cent to prevent the Club being dominated by London-based practitioners and it is suspected that the words "of Great Britain" in the title came to be used at the same time. There is no recorded minute as such. The Army has been represented from the outset, the Club having the Heads of Dental Services in three armed services as members. Sutton Taylor's long association with the Army certainly determined this feature of the membership.

The possibility of publishing the proceedings of the scientific meetings was to be explored, and this is a recurrent matter in the early minutes. However, they were never published, but an offer was made to the Club by John Hovell, the first editor of the British Journal of Oral Surgery in October 1962. Hovell was a Club member, but the papers referred to were those presented to the Club, which were not what Hovell wanted. By 1962 the famous Rule 8, that concerning submissions by Club members, had gone but, to be fair, in the first volume of the British Journal of Oral Surgery (1963) eleven of the twenty-seven contributors were Club members. So the Club was active with its pen as well as its scalpel, but up to that point none of the scientific journals were interested in the Club's offer.

At the end of the meeting at Barnby Moor they decided to change the rule of membership, which was to have a profound effect on the Club. It is minuted:

*It was agreed that the membership of the club be limited to 50 active members and that all candidates for membership must be sponsored by a member and supported by at least two other members. Their election to be carried out at a Meeting of the Club on report by the Committee.*

The significance of this was that the membership was likely to contain most of the leaders of the specialty, the fifteen per cent of movers in any group with a broad membership will have. Not surprisingly the Club and its members have been instrumental in the development of the specialty. However, since its scientific proceedings have never been published, and because of the nature of its membership rule, those outside have often termed it the "mafia". This is not so, as it is not interested in itself as such, but in the furtherance of the science and art of oral surgery. Naturally, there are and have been leaders who have not become members of the Club, but personality is an important element in any small organisation and one or two have dropped out.

Before the Leeds meeting, the Steering Committee met for a third time at the Dental School in Leeds on 17 October 1937. Here it is minuted again over the difficulty in getting the Club's proceedings published. The membership rule was changed for a third time, the pragmatic hand of Sutton Taylor probably behind it. There was to be the category of Honorary Membership, the Committee having the power to elect, and reiterating "That application for Active Membership must have qualifications registerable in this country."

Taylor could see that good links with Europe would be beneficial, and restriction of membership to UK qualifications would exclude any potential members in Europe. The category of Honorary Membership would allow such members, and this has been most important as the club has Honorary Members in several European countries. The category has also allowed active members who have retired from clinical practice to remain members of the Club.

The number of active members on the Committee was increased from two to five. It is likely that Professor Wilkinson, who had been co-opted on to the Committee at the Barnby Moor meeting, wanted to stay on, but co-option would end at the first Annual Meeting when the constitution, being typed before the meeting has the word "four" struck out and substituted with "five". Probably Harold Round and A.E.

Rowlett had already been approached by Taylor before the meeting. When the Club resumed its activities after the War, the number of active Committee Members continued with five, Wilkinson always attending. However, when the Rules were revised in 1949, the number returned to four. After the first Annual General Meeting a better copy of the Rules was typed out but error still crept in, the date being corrected.

The first foreign meeting was considered. The Honorary Secretary was instructed "to explore the possibility of this country (Holland) keeping in mind the best time would be about the end of April." The Club's overseas meetings, by and large, have occurred between March and June. Finally they formally agreed that the first Annual General Meeting of the Club should coincide with the clinical meeting being held by Professor Talmage Read at Leeds on 26 and 27 November 1937, giving Sutton Taylor about a week to inform Club members in sufficient time.

By all accounts this was a prestigious occasion, with eighteen out of the twenty-one members attending the AGM on 26 November. Woods, Young and Hall Fenton were absent for that meeting, but managed to attend the scientific meeting the next day as they appear on the group photograph with Milne, C. Read and Russell Marsh who were elected at that meeting. The original cine clip of that moment taken by Adam Cubie, is in the Club Archive and has been transferred to video tape.

At the Annual General Meeting, the President "......... expressed the hope that goodwill would exist between members and that all petty spite would be absent." He referred to the government of the Club and pointed out "..... that it would be necessary for the Committee to have wide powers." The first sentiment has persisted within the membership of the Club, and is best encapsulated when considering a possible new member by the criterion espoused by Alan Moule: "is he clubbable?" The male "he" will be noted, and the subject of gender is addressed later. However, with the second sentiment, some matters never seem to change.

The Provisional Rules were adopted but, as far as can be ascertained from the records, how long Rule 8, that is, presenting an annual dissertation or case report, existed is not known, but the Second World War was imminent and attitudes had changed by the time hostilities ceased. However, in the early post-war meetings of the Club substantial contributions from members were a feature, and often made up most of the presentations.

The Annual General Meeting was held at 7 p.m. and must have

appeared to be very formal, as they would all be in dinner jackets since the Annual Dinner was scheduled for 8 p.m. This was not a lavish affair but there is no mention on the dinner card as to what was drunk for toasts. Those present at the dinner were told that another prestigious and famous club was founded at Leeds, the Moynihan Surgical Club, and hope was expressed that the Oral Surgery Club would follow the great tradition established.

The Scientific Meeting provided by Professor Talmage Read and his colleagues gives a good insight into the scope and range of practice then. The programme was a mixture of operations, clinical cases and papers:

### *Saturday*

*9 a.m.        Operations*

*(1)    Dental cyst.        Professor Read at Dental School*

*(2)    Cleft palate.        Mr Oldfield at General Infirmary*

*(3)    Arthroplasty of Low Jaw.   Mr Broomhead at General Infirmary*

*Photograph. Outside Dental School*

*Lunch at Staff House*

*Tickets 2/6, exclusive of wine*

*Cases and Discussion at Dental School*

*(1)    Clinical Cases and Operative Results.   Professor Read*

*(2)      Clicking Jaws.   Mr Broomhead*

*(3)      Radium Cases and Cleft Palates.   Mr Oldfield*

*4.00 p.m.      Tea*

*4.30 p.m.      Short papers (10 minutes each)*

*(1)    Calculus of Salivary Glands.        Mr Hamilton Bailey*

*(2)    Agranulocyotosis.        Major Drummond*

*(3)    Hyperastis of Maxilla.        Mr Pain*

*(4)    Osteomyelitis of Mandible.        Mr Taylor*

*(5)    Military Fractures of the Jaw.        Major Woods*

*Concluding Meeting*

*Vote of Thanks*

*Dinner*

**Sunday** *Golf for those who wish.*

Arthroplasty of Low Jaw seems a perplexing title for an operation, but could it have been a modification of the Kostecka operation for a prognathic mandible? In the afternoon the eye alights on Mr Hamilton Bailey's contribution. He was a founder member and was a famous general surgeon at the time, and the author of the seminal book on surgery and based in London. There are two reprints on the subject of salivary glands and calculi written by him in the archives, the first in 1924 for the British Journal of Surgery and the second in 1934 for the Practitioner.

All the other papers were given by Club members. Mr Pain's contribution on Hyperastis of Maxilla was probably a case of hyperostosis. The pattern of this meeting was very similar to what the Club experiences on its visits to foreign centres.

The Annual General Meeting was resumed at 5.30 pm on Saturday 27th November. Votes of thanks were passed, and the Committee reconvened immediately afterwards and proposed a further five names. Some variations to the Rules were beginning to creep in and the pragmatic hands of Sutton Taylor and Talmage Read can be detected. In the list of members there is F.H. Bentley, a plastic surgeon, who was elected at that meeting with C. Read, a radiologist, not oral surgeons but obviously two people with an interest in the subject and who worked and supported oral surgeons. This has been a feature of the Club membership ever since, with the occasional general surgeon, plastic surgeon, orthodontist and pathologist being a member. General surgeons at that time often carried out some oral surgery. F.H. Bentley was elected President of the Club in 1949, and it is quite clear that this was not an inward-looking Organisation as it might appear. They were already prepared for change.

Establishing precisely who the founder members were and those who were elected in the pre-war years has not been easy, as the Minute Book has an incomplete record when compared with the Cash Book. However, the list shown for this period concurs with the number of members given in the Minutes Book and, deducing from written sources, when those members were likely to have been elected.

The Committee next met at Sutton Taylor's house in Portland Place on 26 February 1938 to consider the venue for the foreign meeting.

Holland had already been suggested, but this had appeared not to be possible. Berlin was suggested as an alternative. The Club has always had a spirit of adventure, is not bothered about "heavy fire", and shows initiative. However, at the Annual General Meeting held in Birmingham on 24 June 1938, it is minuted:

> *The Committee has been unable to arrange a meeting abroad because of the uncertain state of foreign affairs and had decided that the Club should meet in England (Birmingham) on this occasion.*

To put matters into historical context, the suggestion of Berlin was made on 26 February 1938. The Austrian Chancellor had just been forced by Hitler to take several Nazis into his Cabinet. On 11 March, just thirteen days after the Club Committee meeting, Austria was forcibly annexed by Hitler, the Anschluss or joining of the two countries. Czechoslovakia was next on the list and Mussolini had already annexed Ethiopia. There were frequent rallies of the SS shouting "Seig Heil", Hail, Victory, and indeed the war clouds were gathering thick and fast over Europe.

A letter to the members from Taylor dated 10 March, the day before the Anschluss, concerning the arrangements for the visit to Berlin is quite clear that detailed provisional arrangements for the visit had been made, together with costing of the trip. However, a further letter dated 12 April 1938, indicated that the meeting was off.

The Minute of the Committee meeting held immediately before the Annual General Meeting of 24 June is a little more explicit. It must be remembered that Sutton Taylor was a commissioned officer in the TA (RAMC) as were several other members, and two were regular serving officers in the Army, Woods and Drummond, the latter becoming a Lt. General. The minute reads:

> *... the Secretary reported that the Berlin meeting suggested at the Committee Meeting of 26 Feb could not be held as several service members found a journey of this nature was not received by the War Office with favour."*

Clearly they had been told that they could not go. Historically, this incident indicates that the War Office was already regarding Germany as hostile, and if they had gone there would have been a high risk of being interned. Chamberlain's famous speech of "Peace in our time" was in the September of that year, and essentially the politicians were trying to buy time in which to modernise the armed forces.

The Club seems to have a penchant for trying to organise meetings in which the country to be visited becomes inappropriate. Some thirty years later another foreign visit was cancelled, because of a revolution this time. A visit to Paris from 5 to 7 June 1968 had been arranged, when at that weekend the Fourth Republic had collapsed following rioting in Paris for the most of May. Jacques Levignanc, the Club's would-be host, in his letter to Ian Heslop, the Secretary, shows almost a British form of sangfroid.

*Paris, le 30 juillet 1968*

*Dear Doctor Heslop*

*The French revolution is over now with many less casualties than in normal time with traffic accidents but with some problems left.*

*I am about to leave for vacations like everybody in Paris which will be for one month a foreign city where all languages are spoken but French. We like that.*

*I must tell you on behalf of Professor AUBRY, Professor CERNEA, Dr DUPUIS, Dr MERVILLE and myself that the Oral Surgery Club will be most welcome in Paris any time.*

*I had a real nice program arranged for the Club it is unfortunate we could not go through but we can do as well next time.*

*Nothing is lost and friendship gained.*

*I send you my best personal regards.*

*Sincerely yours*

*J. Levignac*

So they did, the following year.

Another occasion was the Autumn meeting in Belfast from 26 to 28 October 1977, with Roy Whitlock. This was at the height of the "troubles" and the meeting was held at the Royal Victoria Hospital, which lies besides the Falls Road. There were armed Army personnel patrolling the corridors and grounds of the hospital, helicopters coming and going, and the atmosphere was tense. Whitlock told Club members afterwards that at least half of the waitresses who waited upon the Club at a Reception Dinner were probably linked to the IRA.

Returning to 1938, the Birmingham meeting (the Berlin substitute), the membership stood at thirty-four, the net assets were about £25, and auditors were thought to be necessary. Another member was elected, and the minute ends, "The meeting was then closed to allow the members to enjoy dinner."

The scientific meeting on Saturday 25 June consisted of clinical case presentations by Harold Round and Ralph Broderick, both Club members, in the first half of the morning, with papers in the second half.

*Brief résumé of the diagnosis of Focal Infection.—Professor Wilkinson*

*A Case of Dental Cyst—Mr Russell Marsh*

*After Care of Surgical Cases.—Mr A.M. Nodine*

*A Case of Ulceration of the Tongue- Mr L.M.. Young*

*Localization of Foreign Bodies by X-Rays.- Dr Charles Read*

In the afternoon there were operations by Harold Round, Ralph Broderick and Mr Rainsford Mowlem, who was a plastic surgeon and became the head of the famous Mount Vernon Unit in the Second World War. On the Sunday, they visited a new hospital centre in the morning and visited the local countryside in the afternoon with tea.

A large part of any secretary's job is to chase all manner of items:

*ORAL SURGERY CLUB*

*Number Six*

*88 Portland Place*

*London W.1*

*12th July 1938*

*Dear*

*I would be pleased to receive a cheque for £1.1.0 being your Annual Subscription due July 1st.*

*Also a cheque for    being the amount owing to the Club in respect of the Annual Dinner.*

*I would like to remind you that you have not yet forwarded the compulsory contribution required under the Rules of the Club. This need not be a long article, a comparatively short description of a case will suffice.*

*Yours sincerely*

*R.S. Taylor   Hon Secretary ORAL SURGERY CLUB*

No slacking by members for producing their annual scientific article was being tolerated.

The next meeting was scheduled for Leicester under the Presidency of A.E. Rowlett, who had organised the meeting for 27 and 28 January 1939. Unfortunately, he fell ill and was unable to host the meeting. He was installed as President in absentia, and Professor Talmage Read acted as deputy. At that meeting the Committee considered six more names for membership, but turned one down as he did not fulfil the criteria. The Committee also received the first resignation from the Club, A.M. Milne of Bradford who had been elected two years previously. He found he was unable to attend the meetings, or was it the burden of writing those essays? He made the Leeds meeting, and Leicester was only the third meeting of the Club. However, L. MacLaren Young from Ayr, a founder member submitted two case histories on 14 November 1937, two weeks before the first meeting of the Club. This is the only preserved submission in the archive and the subject is the surgical management of the buried maxillary canine, suitably illustrated. Young had remained a member of the Club for sixty years.

Minuted as another gem. Mr Froggatt of Sheffield had not paid his annual subscription and "...the Committee instructed the Secretary to deal with the matter." Rupert Sutton Taylor was not a man to be trifled with, but there is no record for Froggatt in the Cash Book for 1939. However, he had paid up his guinea in 1947, so he had not been drummed out of the Club and had survived the War.

The scientific programme followed the previous pattern, with operations at Leicester Royal Infirmary followed by clinical cases on the Saturday morning and papers in the afternoon by three members of the Club and one invited speaker. Mr Frizelle demonstrated an operation for hare lip and cleft palate, and in the clinical case presentations showed his results. Cases of adamantinoma of the mandible, malignant tumour of the maxilla, osteomyelitis of the jaw, haemangioma of the tongue, chronic ulcer of the palate (for diagnosis), tumour of the cheek (for diagnosis), cyst of the jaw and necrosis of the alveolus. Cases of jaw fracture. tumours of the submaxillary gland, carcinoma of the antrum, epulis of jaw, carcinoma of ethmoid, lupus of palate and oral leukoplakia were shown. Clearly a very wide range of pathology was seen, the like of which is rarely seen today.

The papers consisted of a case of adamantinoma of the mandible by Professor Roberts and a case of extensive dental sepsis by Hall Fenton. Rowlett was scheduled to give a contribution but, at short notice, S. Hanreck provided a substitute paper on sarcoma. There were two invited speakers, Dr Stewart Johnson, who spoke on malignant tumours of the maxilla, and Dr Van Omen of Holland, on uncommon cases of fractures of the upper and lower jaws.

In the minutes of the Leicester Annual General Meeting, "It was proposed the next meeting of the Club should be abroad." The alternative was Sheffield under Professor Roberts. From copies of the letters in the archive it was clear that the Club wished to visit Paris. Neither meeting was held; war was declared on 4th September and saw some members abroad in a different role. The Honorary Secretary sent out this notice on 7 September:

*Number Six*

*88 Portland Place*

*London, W.1.*

*ORAL SURGERY CLUB*

*Owing to the present situation there will be no meeting in Paris at the end of September.*

*As Major R.S. Taylor is absent on Military Duty, the Funds of the Club, together with a copy of the Rules and a list of names and addresses of the Committee and Members, have been deposited at Westminster Bank, 1, Cavendish Square, London, W.1.*

*7th September 1939*

He had been called up for battle duty.

Perforce, the Club was in a state of suspension until after the War was over, and who knew who would return, particularly the Honorary Secretary who was commanding a Field Ambulance Unit? He did return, unscathed, being awarded an OBE Military Division in recognition of his efforts and being promoted from Major to Lt.Colonel.

There follows a seven-and-a-half year break in proceedings, and it is worth assessing the Club's progress. From Taylor's first concept to the outbreak of War, just three years, the Club had been established. There were thirty-nine members, three scientific meetings had been held, but they had not made it abroad through no fault of theirs. At Leicester in 1939 it is minuted, "The Members continue to show a very keen interest in the wellfair (*sic*) of the Club." The Secretary's spelling showed the slight eccentricity of the man. Taylor should have been well pleased, and the balance sheet stood at £85.8s.1d when the Club's activities were suspended.

Fortunately for oral and maxillofacial surgery all the Club members survived, as did the bank vault in which all the records were held or otherwise the record of the early years could have only been anecdotal. Those who had served in the armed services came back having all been promoted, which augured well for the Club as it began to be involved with the National Health Service Act. This was to change the pattern of delivery of health care in this country and become an even greater catalyst to the advancement of dentistry, and in particular this specialty. War always provides a stimulus, but Aneurin Bevan would surpass that.

The Honorary Secretary's flat had also survived and on 1 November 1946, which must have been soon after his demobilisation, he sent a circular to all Club members announcing the first post-war meeting of the Club at Cheltenham between 28 February and 2 March 1947. Mr A.E. Rowlett remained President, but unfortunately he was ill again and could not go. T. Jackson, who was hosting the meeting, took the chair as Professor Talmage Read, who had deputised before, could not go either. The weather conditions were severe, the infamous winter of 1946/47 had gripped the country but, undaunted, a good turn out of members occurred.

The meeting was held in the Council Chamber of Cheltenham Town Hall, a unique occurrence in the history of the Club. The scientific part of the meeting was held in the morning of Saturday 1 March with the business meeting in the afternoon. There was an informal dinner in the evening, clothes rationing was still in force and perhaps some members were unable to replace their old dinner jackets which no doubt had deteriorated in the War years.

The scientific part of the meeting was devoted to maxillofacial injuries. This is of considerable interest and Kelsey-Fry, who was elected a member at that meeting, had produced in 1942, with others, an important book, *The Dental Treatment of Maxillofacial Injuries*. Interestingly, in the acknowledgements of the book, the authors thank Mrs Lindsay, the BDA librarian for the great help she gave them.

The contributions and the discussion are of interest: pin fixation, a favourite with the American Forces, was thought to have been over used but it certainly had a place in the surgical repertoire, particularly for the edentulous mandible. With the advent of antibiotics, was primary bone grafting now viable? The management of comminuted fractures was discussed. Brigadier Broderick discussed the death rate in maxillofacial injuries, and estimated three per cent succumbed through asphyxia between the Field Ambulance and the Casualty Clearing Station. For A. Pain and Sutton Taylor, in their experience in the forward battle zone, the immediate death rate of maxillofacial injuries was very high and the majority of patients died before reaching the Recovery Ambulance Party. It was impossible to get any figures, but they noted the low death rate after reaching assistance. This reflected great credit on the arrangements for treating maxillofacial injuries. It is of interest that in the First World War, again this was a common experience.

To digress, Pain and Taylor were often at risk of being killed as many in these units were hit. It was the surgical experience gained in these conditions that contributed enormously to the development of the specialty. Those who were not called up worked in the Emergency Medical Service Hospitals, where the war casualties received more definitive and innovative treatment. The Moule pin was developed during this time at Bagueley, Alan Moule turning the prototypes on a lathe himself. He was elected to the Club in June 1948. During the war period, many young maxillofacial surgeons recruited from the dental profession worked with plastic surgeons in the Emergency Medical Service Hospitals. It was there, to a large extent, the real development of the specialty started. Moule worked with Randal Champion, the plastic surgeon, at Bagueley, but equally famous were the three big units in the south of England: Harold Gilles, the plastic surgeon at Basing-stoke, with Norman Rowe and Homer Killey providing the maxillofacial input, McIndoe at East Grinstead with Kelsey-Fry and Ward, and Rainsford Mowlem at Mount Vernon with Ben Fickling giving the maxillofacial support. All these oral surgeons became members of the Club.

To return to the discussions at Cheltenham, there was some debate over the suitability of stainless steel compared with the newer metals such as tantalum.

In the minutes of the Annual General Meeting the following entry appears.

*Consultants Committee. The Secretary reported that he had been in touch with Mr Senior of the BDA as to the need of a consultants committee to advise in connection with the National Health Service Bill. The BDA had taken steps to form such a committee.*

*Proposed by Brig. Broderick and seconded by Mr Davis Thomas that the sec to be instructed to approach the Secretary of the BDA and see what help the Club could give in the matter of the Consultants Committee. Carried.*

The role of the Club was changing from a purely academic pursuit to being a hybrid, showing interest in medical politics as well as to advance the specialty. Given the major change in the climate of practice, involvement of this nature was essential for the specialty to advance.

Five guineas were voted to Miss Snell, Taylor's secretary, which was quite a large sum then; she had no doubt earned it helping Taylor resurrect the Club.

To move forward in time, the offer to the BDA was taken up and Broderick and Taylor were appointed to a sub-committee of the BDA Hospitals Group. Taylor ultimately became the first chairman of the Central Committee of Hospital Dental Consultants and Specialists, the forerunner of the present Central Committee for Hospital Dental Services.

Times were not easy in the early post-war years. From the minute of the Committee meeting of 11 April 1947 it was decided that the Club would hold its first foreign meeting in Holland in early September, lasting four days including travel. The Honorary Secretary ".... was instructed to explore the possibility of obtaining help from the British Council towards the expense of this meeting." One might laugh at this today, but although this country had won the War it was destitute, or nearly so. As Wellington said, "the nearest run thing you ever saw in your life." The request fell on deaf ears, but all the same they went to Utrecht, where by all accounts Dr Tjebbes and his unit put on an impressive meeting between 5 and 7 September 1947. The Club was impressed by the high standard of surgery in the repair of hare lip and cleft palate. Dr Tjebbes was made the first Honorary Member of the Club from overseas. It is of interest that the Club members remain, to this day, impressed at the standard of work in this field on the Continent compared to the results obtained in the UK. Some of the Club's members have been demonstrating an impressive standard of best practice of some years now, using the techniques of Professor Jean Delaire of Nantes (whom the Club visited in 1981) against great opposition.

It became apparent many years later as to why the Club went to Utrecht: why not Paris? On the Club's second visit to Utrecht in 1982, the Honorary Secretary at that time spoke to his old chief for advice as to where in Utrecht the Club could hold its dinner. He was advised to go to the Hotel Pays Bas. Taylor and his men had "liberated" the hotel in 1945 with its wine cellars. The hotel had preserved its guest book, and there was the inimitable handwriting of Taylor at the appropriate place. Needless to say, the Club with their Dutch colleagues had a very memorable evening, as did the hotel staff.

The Club continued to be highly successful, and before long the fifty mark had been reached with more on the "waiting list". The minute of the Annual General Meeting in Manchester on 9 January 1948 makes it clear that the Club had reached this point with the election of nine new members. This was the highest number of active members in the history of the Club until the Annual General Meeting on 2 November 2000, when the number rose to fifty once more. At the 1948 meeting the Rules were revised, and the clause requiring an annual case report or dissertation was dropped. The attendance requirement of at least one meeting in two years was introduced.

The informal nature of the Club had become an important feature, and because it was of a manageable size clinical meetings were a practical feature of all the meetings both home and abroad. It must be appreciated that at the time oral surgery was an emerging specialty. Surgical training and experience was gained from trauma, and correction of facial deformity was an uncommon procedure as deformities were ill-understood. There were a large number of unanswered questions, particularly in the pathology of the region, and the climate that the Club provided was ideal for discussion and debate. Talmage Read's plea at the first Annual General Meeting in 1937, "let there be no spite or pettiness" turned out to be unnecessary: the Club was a very friendly organisation, its members valued each other and a camaraderie existed – hence Weldon Moule's memorable criterion for membership, "is he clubbable?"

After the Utrecht meeting of 1947 came the Manchester meeting, with Professor Frank Wilkinson as President, in January 1948, and the overseas meeting that year was to be in Dublin between 16 and 20 September. At that meeting the members worked hard. The first day, Friday was spent looking at cases of malignant disease and discussing their treatment, first at St Anne's Hospital in the morning and then at the Royal City of Dublin Hospital in the afternoon. That evening the Club entertained the staff of the Incorporated Dental School to dinner. The next day, Saturday, a visit to the Royal College of Surgeons and then on to the famous library in Trinity College, all in the morning.

On Saturday evening the Club members were the guests of the staff of the Incorporated Dental Hospital of Ireland. Sunday was spent in private study and most cases helped by Dublin friends. The members returned to the UK on Monday.

The Secretary did well to remember.

In September 1949 the lack of dinner jackets was becoming a sign of slipping standards and there was no excuse now as clothes rationing had ceased on 15 March. "It was decided to recommend to members that dinner jackets be worn at Club dinners in future." And they have ever since.

The life of an Honorary Secretary is not always a happy one. The minute of the Committee meeting at Leeds on 19 December 1953 is brief, even for a man who believed in brevity and who demanded that his juniors read Sir Ernest Gower's book *Plain Words*.

*It has proved difficult to report this meeting in greater detail because the Sec. has lost his notes of this meeting, they are believed to have been left in the train.*

It can happen to us all.

Looking at the scientific programmes, those at the home meetings continued in much the same format with sometimes operative technique being demonstrated but usually clinical case presentations and lectures given on related topics. The members were still involved, but they often came from either the unit of the President for the year or a nearby unit or hospital. The emphasis of the subjects covered has changed and at the same time the Club has seen an amazing development and growth of the specialty, so much so that it is seen as part of the surgical spectrum, which in reality it is, albeit specialised as is dentistry an important part of the health care. As mentioned previously, the broad nature of the home programmes is important educationally and they are recognised as such. The problem with any specialisation is that it becomes narrow in outlook very easily unless deliberate steps are taken to avoid it.

The overseas meetings show little change in pattern and content. On average some twenty members attend, but the number has been as high as thirty-five plus spouses. These numbers are manageable which maintains the nature and character of these meetings, and are recognised as part of continuing medical education, a role the Club has played since its inception. The Club has only strayed outside Europe twice, once to New York in September 1949 when only three members went, and recently to Israel in 2000. In the spirit of adventure, they went behind the Iron Curtain to Prague in 1973. An eminent member of the Club was arrested as the driver for allegedly driving round a roundabout the wrong way late at night. He was, in fact, the front seat passenger in the

Honorary Secretary's right hand drive minibus.

In 1985 the Club went behind the Iron Curtain again, this time to Budapest to the unit of Professor Georgi Szabo. This was a highly successful meeting, with the clinical day starting at 7 a.m. with a glass of Schnapps! The Honorary Secretary at the time had quickly concluded that the "guide" allotted to the party by the Government Tourist Office, which controlled all tourism, was really from the Ministry for the Interior. When confronted with this deduction, the guide was quickly reassured that the Club did not pose a security risk and as a result she ensured the very smooth running of the visit. The Club was granted a most notable award by the Semmelweis University of Medicine of Budapest – the Semmelweis Medal, a rare honour. An early recipient was Nikita Khrushchev, and the Club's medal was No 19. With a gift such as this for an organisation with no fixed base, placing it in its box and leaving it in some drawer would result in its loss. As the President had no Presidential insignia, the medal was mounted in silver and is worn proudly by every President since. Semmelweis was the first person to realise that the cause of Puerperal sepsis in post partum women in the late nineteenth century was caused by cross infection arising from poor hygiene practised by the doctors. They failed to wash their hands thoroughly between the post mortem room and examining their patients. Puerperal sepsis in those days was usually fatal. He was ostracised by his outraged colleagues, but ultimately his findings were accepted. Admitting to wrong practice has usually been difficult and remains difficult for some.

During its history, the Club has visited forty-three units abroad, most frequently to France, Holland, Belgium, Austria and Switzerland, but it still has not been to Berlin, its first choice for 1938. Members find these visits of great benefit, which is translated into patient care provided by them.

Reviewing the minutes over the years, the subject of membership continues to emerge at various times. In June 1978, it had fallen to thirty-four active members and seventeen honorary members, which is the lowest it has been since January 1948. Since then the figure fluctuates with an upward trend, and today the membership is full with fifty active members and fifty-two honorary members. The subject of women taking part in the meetings, let alone becoming members, has been a delicate affair as the Club was perceived as being an all-male organisation. At the Edinburgh meeting in March 1950 it is minuted "All persons (not being members of the Club), who demonstrate to the Club or read papers to the Club should be Club guests." The President for the year at his meeting in Canterbury was concerned that, because of this perception, he would not be able to bring one of his lecturers, a very eminent person in her field, to the Club dinner. He was advised that there was no difficulty. After all the Club, in its 50th Anniversary Year in 1987, went to Salzburg to Professor Helene Matras' unit, another highly successful meeting. The question as to why the Club appears not to have any women members arises. Firstly, there are very few women consultants in the specialty, which mitigates against them becoming members. However, two highly distinguished women were elected members at the Annual General Meeting in November 2000. Speculation as to what the founders of the Club might have felt with these elections is intriguing, but they probably would have reacted favourably. The conceptor, Rupert Sutton Taylor, was the first consultant oral surgeon to have a woman senior registrar, Isobelle Thompson, in 1961. He was ribbed by some of his illustrious colleagues as might be imagined, but she became the first woman regional consultant oral surgeon in the UK, being appointed to Eastbourne. Alan Weldon Moule was another who, shortly after had Miss Nina Shotts as his senior registrar, and she became consultant at the West Middlesex Hospital.

The Club has changed in subtle ways: geographical spread has always been important, and any London domination was countered by the twenty-five per cent rule. Looking at the present list, the distribution is fairly even across the country and reflects the population distribution. The distribution pattern of the whole membership since the Club's inception is very similar to that of the current membership, both active and honorary. As for London, only three of the fifty active members and five of the fifty-two honorary members represent the Capital, just eight per cent in all. This is the result of amalgamation of so many hospitals and the inevitable reduction in the numbers of consultant staff. It would seem that a London-based dominance is highly unlikely.

So, are the Club members playing crucial roles in the specialty and dentistry? The answer is a most affirmative "yes". They are involved in all spheres of education and training including the Universities, they are amongst the advisors to Government, they are involved with the British Dental Association at many levels and they are involved often at a high level with European professional associations. Are they advancing the science and art of oral surgery? Again, most certainly, yes. The names of members are regularly in the published scientific literature and figure prominently in the annual scientific programmes of the British Association of Oral and Maxillofacial Surgeons.

In 1962, Rupert Sutton Taylor decided that he had made his contribution and retired from the secretaryship of the Club, and the following year handed over the treasurership after twenty-five years fulfilling the dual post. He was made President the following year. However, also in 1962, the British Association of Oral and Maxillofacial Surgeons was founded with Taylor and some Club members on the Steering Committee. In his speech to the Club when standing down from the secretaryship in Ipswich on 18 October, which was recorded on tape, he thought that the Club's purpose would fade with the advent of the new specialty association: the Club would be eclipsed. He thought that the Club would become just a very exclusive dining club. He was correct about most things, but with this he was wrong. The two organisations fulfil two very different purposes and 45 years after that speech, the Oral Surgery Club of Great Britain is thriving and 70 years young, and is still at the cutting edge.

John Bradley May 2001

# 2011 update.

In the 75th Anniversary Year of its inception, an update of the History of the Oral Surgery Club of Great Britain seems appropriate.

In the early years of the Club, there were a few active members outside the field of Oral Surgery, who none the less had an interest in the subject. They came from the fields of general surgery, plastic surgery, orthodontics and radiology. As the Club was a very new institution, their presence was thought to be advantageous. However, such a spectrum of membership was felt to be no longer necessary and in 2002 it was decided that membership should come from within the specialty of oral and maxillofacial surgery. There was one UK honorary member who would no longer fulfil this requirement but it was unanimously agreed that he should remain an honorary member.

The membership (2007) remains at near its maximum level with 48 active members and 57 honorary members. Over the last few years there has been a trend, albeit a small but noticeable number of people who have not accepted the invitation to join the Club. There is also a noticeable number who have accepted but failed to attend any of the meetings thus allowing their membership to lapse. Perhaps they are too busy and you cannot join all the specialty associations. However, the Club continues to attract members who are clearly foremost in the specialty.

The destinations of overseas visits are largely European but the Club is being more adventurous visiting New York (2005) and Houston (2009), looking East, it went to Muscat in 2010 and is planning to go back to the USA in 2012 to Baltimore. With the huge populations in the Far East, there is vibrant activity within our specialty as can be seen from the papers published in the scientific journals of the West. Perhaps a visit would be a memorable experience: one of our number regularly goes to India to teach the repair of cleft lip and palate, but managing a different and challenging pathology is another matter. Some recognition of the giving rather than the taking (CME points) with more senior colleagues by our Regulatory Bodies is long overdue.

Overseas meetings are popular and are well attended (22 to 30). Our colleagues always organise excellent informative meetings and the benefit of this, when translated to practice in the UK, is most valuable for the patient. Subjects range from head and neck malignancy and reconstruction, the correction of facial deformity including cleft lip and palate, skull base surgery, trauma, endoscopic approach to obstructive salivary gland disease and sinus disease, numerous research projects from bio-materials to clinical programmes. Many of these programmes include theatre sessions and out patient clinics to see the results of treatment, an activity sadly impossible to do in the present NHS.

The home meetings have all been well attended and, following tradition, the majority of subjects are outside the specialty. They have all provoked lively discussion and much is learnt. Most people's practice impinges on many of the subjects presented and discussed and members are always grateful for those invited to give papers.

Continuing Medical Education (CME) has been a major part of the Club's raison d'être but in these formalised bureaucratic times every active practitioner has to clock up a minimum number of points per annum. The Club's meetings are "valued" and CME points awarded. For example, the Club visit to Dr Danny Temkin's unit at Poriya, Israel, was awarded 9 points. However, the meeting to Professor Devauchelle's unit at Amiens was considered to be more beneficial and was awarded 14 points. Home meetings are, by and large, poorly awarded: the assessors fail to grasp the point that to receive a rounded education, a narrow experience will not provide it.

In 2000 the members were asked for their views on the format of the meetings and whether changes were desirable since the pattern had remained unaltered for 25 years. A large majority were satisfied with the existing format and advocated no change but with regard to the overseas meetings, 13 members felt a full two day meeting was preferable but 26 thought that the pace would be too hot and suggested three half days! However, these meetings are organised by the host unit and the pattern is dependent on their stamina. For example, in 2005 the Club ventured for the second time to New York, the last time being in 1959 when about 6 people attended. This time there was an excellent turn out of 22 members with 16 partners! Professor Jatin Shah had organised a superb meeting conducted at a lively pace from 8.00 a.m. to 5.00 p.m. with a dinner. The following morning there was a 7.30 a.m. start, members demonstrated great stamina and ended the day by entertaining Professor

Shah and his unit to dinner where 52 people sat down.

The Honorary Treasurer has reported over the years a consistently favourable bank balance but at the AGM in November 2000 he noted that the annual subscription of £10.00 had remained unaltered for 12 years. He noted also that the secretarial assistance both he and the Honorary Secretary had received from their own secretaries had, in reality, been poorly remunerated and the position would be untenable. The annual subscription was raised to £25.00 so that the respective secretaries could be paid £300.00 per annum but in November 2003 it was noted that the remuneration of the Honorary Secretary's secretary should be increased to £500.00 per annum in recognition of the considerable amount of work she had undertaken. However, the Honorary Treasurer's secretary remuneration would remain at £300.00 per annum. At least the Committee was now regularly reviewing the position.

Sponsorship to the home meetings by surgical supply and drug companies has been generous over the last ten years given the small size of the Club. The financial contribution made has significantly helped the finances of the club for which the Club remains forever grateful. The costs of the Autumn meeting have become significant and the healthy finances have made it possible for the President of the year to receive a float ahead of the meeting.

The Honorary Treasurer, Peter Banks, stepped down in November 2006 after 20 years in the post having managed the Club's financial affairs most expertly. As with all organisations, he has had his moments chasing up a small number of people who remained consistently in arrears! However, his parting "gift" to the club was that the 70th Anniversary Dinner in Newcastle was paid entirely out of the funds so expertly accrued over the previous 20 years.

The vexed question whether spouses/partners of members should be able to attend the Annual Dinner was raised at the AGM in November 2000. A questionnaire was circulated to all members seeking their opinion and at the AGM of the following year it was reported that the majority view was that the traditional dinner should continue with members only with the presenters of the scientific papers at that meeting as guests of the Club. However, the matter was raised again in 2005 and a debate ensued with Bill Simpson proposing the status quo, that is, members only with guests who had taken part in the scientific part of the President's meeting attending. Richard Juniper gave the opposing argument, both submitted papers for circulation amongst the membership and a postal ballot was to be arranged. At the 2006 AGM a small majority of the members opposed the motion to keep the status quo which meant that the spouses and partners of members could be invited to the Annual Dinner. Tradition dies hard and it will be interesting to see if this new rule has any effect on the character of the Club. On the present evidence, the future of the Club is not in doubt. As noted in the main history of the club, it fulfils a different purpose from that of the main specialty associations.

JCB, August 2011

# Club Members 1937 - 2015

1936   Rupert Sutton-Taylor (Conceptor and Secretary) London

1937   Members of steering committee: Professor T. Talmage-Read (First Chairman 1936/37-Leeds) S.H. Woods-Army, T Hall Fenton-Grimsby, Professor F C Wilkinson-Manchester.

Other members of first committee: Harold Round-Birmingham, A E Rowlett-Leicester.

Other founding members: JSH Collinge-Southport, D Fyle-Glasgow, Hamilton Bailey (Gen. Surg.)-London, J D Cambrook-London, H E Barker-Liverpool, A Cubie-Glasgow, L M Young-Ayr, A Pain-Folkestone, G Froggatt-Sheffield, A E Meeson-Liverpool, A Drummond (Maj.)-Army, A M Nodine-London, L.S.Hanreck-Horsham.

Elected members:

1937 (November) Professor G I Roberts-Sheffield, Professor H H Stones-Liverpool, A M Milne- Bradford, T Jackson-Cheltenham, F H Bentley (Plastic Surgeon) -Manchester, C Read (Radiologist)-Glasgow, H Selby-Brown-London, J Vidler-Windsor, L Russell Marsh-London, Mr Oldfield (Gen. Surg.)-Leeds

1938   J Hayes-?, L Gibson-Kilmarnock, E A Hardy-London, R A Broderick-Birmingham,

1939 D S Middleton-Edinburgh, R O Walker-Birmingham, C D Farris- Cambridge, T G Scott (Pathologist)-Glasgow, Davis Thomas-Birmingham.

1947 W Kelsey Fry-London, Ernest White-London, Professor R

Bradshaw- Newcastle, J T Woods (Surg. Capt.)-Navy

1948  A W Moule-Manchester, L K H Benson-Manchester, T G Ward- Hastings, T Craddock-Henry-London, G Macphee-Liverpool, Professor A D Hitchen-Dundee, Professor J Boyes-Newcastle, B St J Steadman- London, R Cocker-London.

1949  Professor A J Darling-Bristol, F G Gibb-Edinburgh.

1950  B V Janes- Manchester, G Fitzgibbon (Plastic Surg.)-Bristol.

1951   G Hankey-London, J Snawdon-Bristol, F T Monks-Bolton, D C Paley-Battersea (Group Capt.)-Royal Air Force.

1952 No elections.

1953 B S Fickling-Northwood.

1954 No elections.

1955 R Battle (Plastic Surg.)-London.

1956 Professor I R H Kramer-London, C V Taylor (Brig.)-Army, Professor Alec McGregor-Birmingham.

1957 J H Hovell-London.

1958 No elections.

1959 H M Crombie-Aberdeen, D Downton-London, V E Ireland-Ipswich, Professor G L Howe-Newcastle, F G Hardman-Rhyll, R Whitlock-Belfast, Professor H G Radden-Manchester.

1960 H P Cook-London, I H Heslop-Woking.

1961 P A Bramley-Plymouth, W D Maclennan-Edinburgh, D Penney-Bradford, N L Rowe-Roehampton, G M Warrack-Edinburgh.

1962 N Hogan-Dublin.

1963 E J R Morgan-Swansea, Professor H C Killey-London, R O'Neil-London.

1964   J R V B Gibson-Chepstow, B Hales-Stoke, W R Roberts-Worcester.

1965  H M Alty-Liverpool, T G Battersby-Nottingham, P James-London.

1966  No elections

1967  P Bradnum-Newcastle, D Hayton-Williams-Oxford, P H

Burke (Orthodontist)-Cambridge, Professor E D Farmer-Liverpool, G S Hoggins- Birmingham.

1968   P H D Lewars-Exeter.

1969   Professor D Poswillo-London, J H Robertson (Maj. Gen.)-Army.

1970   No elections.

1971   No elections

1972   M D Awty-East Grinstead, A F Hamilton-Cheltenham, G L Manning-Stoke, W Simpson-Manchester.

1973  R L G Dawson (Plastic Surg.)-London, P A Toller-Northwood.

1974   J C Bradley-Burnley, T I English-London, J Rayne-Oxford.

1975   T C Crewe-Plymouth, W Gray-Ipswich, M S Jones-Wolver-hampton, D S Smith-Canterbury, G Smith (Brig.)-Army.

1977   No elections.

1978 Professor G R Seward-London, P R Barton-Oxford, K R Ray-Reading,

A J Quant-(G. Capt.)-Royal Air Force. J M Gorman-Belfast, D Wilson-London.

1980   Professor D A McGowan-Glasgow, J Ll Williams-Chichester.

1981   No elections.

1982   P Selwyn-Nottingham, D A Mason-Bradford.

1983   B D G Morgan (Plastic Surg.)-London, A J Sear-Worcester, G T Cheney-Norwich.

1984   T G Emerson-Londonderry.

1985   T J C Hall (Surg.Capt.)-Navy, Professor P F Bradley-Edinburgh, M J Newell (Brig,).-Army

1986   P J Leopard-Stoke, R P Ward-Booth-Sunderland, C W Rowse-Swansea, M J C Wake-Birmingham.

1987   P G McAndrew-Rotherham, J D W Barnard-Portsmouth.

1988   M E Foster-Manchester, L Oldham-Taunton, R P Juniper-Oxford.

1989   K F Moos-Glasgow.

1990   J E Hawkesford-Newcastle, J C Lowry-Bolton, G A Wood-North Wales, R J Tate-Ipswich, D O Matthews (Air C'dore)-Royal Air Force.

1991   B S Avery-Middlesbrough, J I Cawood-Chester, K M Lavery-West Midland, A F Markus-Poole, A V Babajews-Exeter.

1992   B M W Bailey-Roehampton, M Corrigan-Leeds, D R James-London, R A Smart (Brig.)-Army, E D Vaughan-Liverpool.

1993   S F Olley-Shrewsbury, R W Kendrick-Belfast, M T Simpson-Luton.

1994   J F Hamlyn-Taunton, B G Millar-West Midlands, D W Patton-Swansea.

1995   A E Brown-East Grinstead, T W Negus (Air C'dore)-Royal Air Force,  P J Weller-Southend.

1996   Professor J W Frame-Birmingham.

1997   K Jones-Derby, G Lello-Edinburgh, D Macpherson-Chichester.

1998   J S Brown-Liverpool, I Hutchinson-London, Professor M McGurk-London. G Zaki-Portsmouth.

1999   L F A Stassen-Sunderland, R Woodwards-Manchester, B T Evans- Southampton, A W Sugar-Swansea.

2000   M E Morton-Blackburn, S E Fisher-Leeds, N Baker-Southampton, C Beirne-Dublin, S Dover-Birmingham, J Hayter-Leicester, I H McVicar-Nottingham, T Mellor-Portsmouth, P Ramsay-Baggs-Dundonald, N C Renny-Aberdeen.

2001   D M Adlam-Cambridge.

2002   J Herold-Brighton, I C Martin-Sunderland, A G Smythe-Leeds.

2004   L Newman-London, A G Sadler-Lincoln, A R C Boyd-Londonderry, G J Kearns-Limerick.

2005   C J Kerawala-Basingstoke, D A Koppel-Glasgow ,A J Lyons-London, G D Putnam-Carlisle, J E Rowson-Nottingham, P D Earle-Worcester.

2006   A McLean-Exeter. M Gilhooly-London, D Bryant-Middlesborough.

2007   S Hislop-Glasgow, S Langton-Manchester, A Monaghan-Birmingham.

2008  M Fardy-Cardiff, I Downie-Salisbury, C Pratt-Chichester, A Stewart-London, M Davison-Taunton.

2009  K Webster-Birmingham, A Cronin-Cardiff, D Godden-Cheltenham, P Magennis-Liverpool.

2010  B Visavadia-Harrow, P Ramchandani-Poole.

2011  A Baldwin-Manchester, S Holmes-London, P Revington-Bristol, H Witherow-London

2012 K Altman-Brighton, A Smith-Sheffield, K Sneddon-East Grinstead, B Swinson-Londonderry

2013 M Amin- Harrow, R Anand-Portsmouth, R Bentley-London, D Dhariwal-Oxford, D Laugharne-Derby, C Newlands-Guildford, S Parmar-Birmingham, T Patterson-Rotherham, E Thomson-Forth Valley, S Whitley-London, A Yousefpour-Sheffield

2014 S Sharma-Southampton, C Hughes-Bristol, C Jones-Liverpool, M Kumar-Hillingdon, P Norris- East Grinstead, A Dickenson-Derby, M Heliotis-Northwick Park.

2015 Malcolm Cameron, Mark Devlin, Chetan Katre, Neil Mackenzie, Steven Walsh. .

2016 Martin Paley, Andrew Burns, Victoria Beale, Dilip Srinivasan.

2017 Hazel Busby-Earle Leicester, Jacob D'Souza Guildford, Kathy Fan Kings, Peyman Alam Chichester.

2018  Satheeth Prabhu Oxford, Ajay Wilson Sunderland, Panos Kyzas Manchester, Mo Shorafa Wexham Park.

2019 Mike Essen Exeter, Geoff Chiu Blackburn, Leo Vassiliou Manchester,

# Overseas Honorary Members

1949 Dr J Tjebbes-Utrecht.

1966 Professor H Obwegeser-Zurich.

1970 Professor R Becker-Munster.

1972 Professor C A Merks-Nijmegan,

1976 Professor R Mayer-Brussels.

1981 Professor P Egyedi-Utrecht.

1988 Professor H D Pape-Cologne.

1992 Professor B Gattinger-Linz.

1993 Professor H Sailer-Zurich.

1997 Professor E Machtens-Bochum,

2001 Professor B Deveauchelle-Amiens.

2002 Professor R Schmelzeisen-Freiburg.

2003 Professor R Ewers-Vienna.

2004 Professor S Reinart-Tubingen.

2005 Professor J Shah-New York

2007 Professor T Kreusch-Hamburg.

2008 Professor R Brusati-Milam.

2009 Professor M Wong-Houston.

2010 Dr Mohamed Al Ismaily-Muscat.

2011 Dr H Schliephake-Göttingen

2012 Dr B Ord - Baltimore

# Club Office Holders 1937 - 2021

## Presidents

| | | |
|---|---|---|
| 1937 | Professor T. Talmage Read | Leeds |
| 1938 | Professor T. Talmage Read | Leeds |
| 1939 | A.E. Rowlett | Leicester |
| 1947 | A.E. Rowlett | Leicester |
| 1948 | Professor F.C. Wilkinson | Manchester |
| 1949 | F.H. Bentley | Manchester |
| 1950 | D.S. Middleton | Edinburgh |
| 1951 | Professor H.H. Stones | Liverpool |
| 1952 | A. Cubie | Glasgow |
| 1953 | Col. R.A. Broderick | Birmingham |
| 1954 | Professor T Talmage Read | Leeds |
| 1955 | Professor F.C. Wilkinson | London |
| 1956 | Professor A.D. Hitchen | Dundee |
| 1957 | C.D.Farris | Cambridge |
| 1957/8 | Maj. Gen. A. Drummond | Army |
| 1959 | A.W. Moule | Manchester |
| 1960 | Professor A.I. Darling | Bristol |
| 1961 | T.G. Scott | Glasgow |
| 1962/63 | A. Pain | Folkestone |
| 1963/64 | R.S. Taylor | London |
| 1964/65 | Professor G.L. Howe | Newcastle |
| 1965/66 | J.H. Hovell | London |
| 1966/67 | J.D. Cambrook | London |
| 1967/68 | T.C. Henry | London |
| 1968/69 | Air C'dore D.C. Paley-Battersea | Royal Air Force |
| 1969/70 | R.O. Walker | Birmingham |
| 1970/71 | F.T. Monks | Bolton |
| 1971/72 | J.S.H. Collinge | Southport |
| 1972/73 | F.G. Hardman | Rhyl |
| 1973/74 | B.W. Fickling | Northwood |
| 1974/75 | I.H. Heslop | Guildford |
| 1975/76 | Maj. Gen. J.H. Robertson | Army |
| 1976/77 | D. Downton | London |
| 1977/78 | R. Whitlock | Belfast |
| 1978/79 | J.R.V.B. Gibson | Chepstow |

| Year | Name | Location |
|---|---|---|
| 1979/80 | H.P. Cook | London |
| 1980/81 | D. Penney | Bradford |
| 1981/82 | E.J.R. Morgan | Swansea |
| 1982/83 | W.D. Maclennan | Edinburgh |
| 1983/84 | P.H.D. Lewars | Exeter |
| 1984/85 | H.M. Alty | Liverpool |
| 1985/86 | Professor Sir Paul Bramley | Sheffield |
| 1986/87 | G.L. Manning | Stoke |
| 1987/88 | P. James | London |
| 1988/89 | D.C. Smith | Canterbury |
| 1989/90 | T.C. Crewe | Plymouth |
| 1990/91 | W. Gray | Ipswich |
| 1991/92 | P.B. Clarke | Aberdeen |
| 1992/93 | D. Henderson | London |
| 1993/94 | J.C. Bradley | Burnley |
| 1994/95 | W. Simpson | Manchester |
| 1995/96 | G.T. Cheney | Norwich |
| 1996/97 | J. Ll. Williams | Chichester |
| 1997/98 | C.W. Rowse | Swansea |
| 1998/99 | K.F. Moos | Glasgow |
| 1999/00 | R.P. Juniper | Oxford |
| 2000/01 | P.G. McAndrew | Rotherham |
| 2001/02 | M.E Foster | Alderley Edge |
| 2002/03 | R.J Tate | Ipswich |
| 2003/04 | S.F Olley | Shrewsbury |
| 2004/05 | B.M.W.Bailey | Egham |
| 2005/06 | R. Kendrick | Belfast |
| 2006/07 | J. Hawkesford | Newcastle |
| 2007/08 | A F Markus | Bournemouth |
| 2008/09 | G Wood | Glasgow |
| 2009/10 | M Simpson | Bedford |
| 2010/11 | K Lavery | East Grinstead |
| 2011/12 | D Adlam | Cambridge |
| 2012/13 | P Ramsay-Baggs | Belfast |
| 2013/14 | J Herold | Brighton |
| 2014/15 | M Gilhooly | Northwick Park |
| 2015/16 | Tim Mellor | Portsmouth |
| 2016/17 | Iain McVicar | Nottingham |

| 2017/18 | Stuart Hislop | Glasgow |
| 2018/19 | Phillip Earl | Worcester |
| 2019/21 | Andrew Baldwin | Manchester |
| 2021/22 | Ken Sneddon | East Grinstead |

## Hon Secretaries

| 1937-1963 | R S Taylor, |
| 1963-1974 | I H Heslop |
| 1974-1983 | R O'Neil |
| 1983-1990 | J C Bradley |
| 1990-2000 | M E Foster |
| 2000-2003 | A E Babajews |
| 2003-2006 | R Woodwards |
| 2006-2009 | A Sadler |
| 2009-2011 | A Lyons |
| 2011- 2015 | T Mellor |
| 2015 - | J Hayter |

## Hon Treasurers

| 1937-1963 | R S Taylor, |
| 1963-1986 | D Downton |
| 1986-2006 | P Banks |
| 2006-2009 | K Lavery |
| 2010- | A E Brown |

## Hon Archivists

| 1980-1988 | A W Moule | 1999-2011 | J C Bradley |
| 1988-1999 | D Downton | 2011 - | A Sadler |

# Scientific Meetings  1937 - 2015

1937: Leeds 26-28 Nov
Talmage Read
1938: Berlin cancelled
1938 : Birmingham 24-25 June
Talmage Read
1939: Leicester 27-28 Jan Rowlett
1947: Cheltenham 28 Feb-2 March
Rowlett
1948: Utrecht 4-8 Sept Rowlett
1948: Manchester 9-10 Jan
Wilkinson
1948: Dublin 17-20 Sept Wilkinson
1949: Newcastle 25-26 March
Bentley
1949 Bristol 23-25 Sept Bentley
1950: Edinburgh 30 March-2 April
Middleton
1950: London 27-28 October
Middleton
1951: Liverpool 13-14 April Stones
1952: Paris .24-28 October Stones
1952: Glasgow 24-27 April Cubie
1953: London 29 November Cubie
1953: Birmingham 24-25 April
Broderick
1953: Leeds 17-19 June
Talmage Read
1954: Brussels 3-7 June
Talmage Read
1954: No UK meeting
1955:.London 14-15 Jan Wilkinson
1955: Copenhagen 11-15 Aug
Wilkinson
1956: Dundee 22-24 Jan Hitchen
1956: Groningen 27-30 Sept Hitchen
1957: Cambridge 3-14 April Farris
1957: London 25-26 Oct Drummond
1958: Zurich 16-19 Oct Drummond
1958: No UK meeting
1959: Manchester 1-2 May Moule
1959: New York Sept Moule
1960:.Bristol 28-30 Jan Darling
1960: No overseas meeting
1961: Madrid 27 April-1 May
Darling

1961:  Belfast 19-21 Oct Scott
1962: Ipswich 18-20 Oct Pain
1962: No overseas meeting
1963: Vienna 3-6 April Pain
1963: London 26-27 Oct Taylor
1964: Lisbon 8-11 April Taylor
1964: Newcastle 24-26 Sept Howe
1965: Lyons 21-24 April Howe
1965: London 18-20 Sept Hovell
1966: Zurich 14-17 April Hovell
1966: Plymouth 9-11 June Cambrook
1967: No overseas meeting
1967: London 9-10 Nov Henry
1968: Paris cancelled
1968: London & Farnborough 7-8 Nov
Paley-Battersea
1969:  Paris 21-23 May Paley-Battersea
1969:  Birmingham 6-8 Nov Walker
1970: Munster 24-27 June Walker
1970 Bolton 22-23 Oct Monks
1971: Oslo 5-8 May Monks
1971: Southport 21-22 Oct Collinge
1972: Nijmegan 24-27 May Collinge
1972: Rhyll 26-28 Oct Hardman
1973: Prague 30 May-2 June Hardman
1973 Northwood 25-27 Oct Fickling
1974: No overseas meeting
1974: Guildford 31 Oct– 1 Nov Heslop
1975: Bordeaux 25-30 May Heslop
1975 Aldershot 30-31 Oct Robertson
1976: Brussels 3-4 June Robertson
1976: London 29-2 9Oct Downton
1977: Dublin 30 June-1 July Downton
1977: Belfast 26-28 Oct Whitlock
1978: London 29-30 June Whitlock
1978: Chepstow 26-27 Oct Gibson
1979: Nancy 31 May 1st June Gibson
1979: London 25-26 Oct Cook
1980: Freiburg 2-3 June Cook
1980: Bradford 23-24 Oct Penney
1981: Nantes 6-7 May Penney
1981: Swansea 29-30 Oct Morgan
1982: Utrecht 6-7 May Morgan
1982: Edinburgh 28-29 Oct Maclennan
1983: Munster 5-6 May Maclennan
1983: Exeter 27-28 Oct Lewars

1984: Strasbourg 11-12 April Lewars
1984: Liverpool 1-2 Nov Alty
1985: Budapest 13-14 June Alty
1985: Sheffield 31 Oct-1 Nov Bramley
1986: Nijmegan 24-25 April Bramley
1986: Stoke 30-31 Oct Manning
1987: Salzburg 25-26 March Manning
1987: London 29-30 Oct James
1988: Cologne 2-3 June James
1988: Canterbury 27-28 Oct Smith
1989: Athens 11-12 May Smith
1989: Plymouth 26-27 Oct Crewe
1990: Montpelier 17-18 May Crewe
1990: Ipswich 25-26 Oct Gray
1991: Parma 2-3 May Gray
1991: Aberdeen 31Oct-1 Nov Clarke
1992: Linz 4-5 June Clarke
1992: London 12-13 Nov Henderson
1993: Zurich 5-7 June Henderson
1993: Burnley 4-5 November Bradley
1994: Helsinki 19-20 May Bradley
1994: Manchester 3-4 Nov Simpson
1995: Brugge 3-6 May Simpson
1995: Norwich 2-3 Nov Cheney
1996: Leipzig 16-18 May Cheney
1996: Chichester 7-8 Nov Williams
1997: Bochum 16-19 April Williams
1997: Swansea 6-7 Nov Rowse
1998: Madrid 6-9 May Rowse
1998: Glasgow 12-13 Nov Moos
1999: Amsterdam 6-7 May Moos
1999: Oxford 4-5 Nov Juniper
2000: Israel 24-26 May Juniper
2000: Rotherham 2-3 Nov McAndrew
2001: Amiens 10-11 May McAndrew
2001: Macclesfield 1-2 Nov Foster
2002: Freiburg 15-17 May Foster
2002: Ipswich 31 Oct-1 Nov Tate
2003: Vienna 23-25 April Tate
2003: Shrewsbury 6-7 Nov Olley
2004: Tubingen 13-15 May Olley
2004: Egham 25-26 Nov Bailey
2005: New York 12-14 May Bailey
2005: Belfast 17-19 Nov Kendrick
2006: Groningen 17-19 May Kendrick
2006: Newcastle 16-18 Nov
Hawkesford
2007: Hamburg 2-5 May Hawkesford

2008: Bournemouth 15-17 Nov Markus
2008: Milan 15-16 May Markus
2008: Glasgow 13-14 Nov Wood
2009: Houston 30 April-4 March Wood
2009: Bedford 4-5 Nov Simpson
2010: Muscat 28 Feb-4 March Simpson
2010: East Grinstead 4-5 Nov Lavery
2011: Göttingen 11-13 May Lavery
2011: Cambridge 10-11 Nov Adlam
2012: Belfast 9-10 Nov Ramsay-Baggs
2013: Ferrara 8-10 May Ramsay-Baggs
2013: Brighton 7-9 Nov Herold
2014: Prague 24-25 April Herold
2014 Chesham 6-7 Nov Gilhooly
2015 Salzburg 30 April-May 1$^{st}$ Gilhooly
2015 Old Thorns Liphook Nov 5-6 Mellor
2016 Madrid 5-6 May Mellor
2016 Nottingham Nov 10-11 McVicar
2017 Bangalore May 22-23 McVicar
2017 Troon Nov 2-3 Hislop
2018 Halifax May 16-19 Hislop
2018 Worcester Nov8-9 Earl
2019 Lille May 16-17 Earl
2019 Manchester Nov 7-8 Baldwin

# Rules of the Club

1       That the CLUB be known as the ORAL SURGERY CLUB OF GREAT BRITAIN.

2       That the objects of the CLUB be to advance the Science and Art of Oral and Maxillofacial Surgery.

3       That membership be of two kinds, Active and Honorary

4       a). That Active Membership be open to those appointed to an NHS consultant post in Oral and Maxillofacial Surgery of at least 6 sessions (or equivalent in the University or Armed Services). Any subsequent reduction of sessions will not affect active membership status. Hence, independent practice or non-clinical NHS work such as Trust Chair would not affect the above.

        b). Active members shall become Honorary members on reaching the age of 65 or on stopping all professional practice whichever is the earlier.

5       That all persons desiring to become Active Members be required to satisfy the Committee that they are eligible under Rule four. Candidates for membership must be sponsored by a member and supported by at least two other members. Their election will be carried out at a meeting of the CLUB on report by the Committee.

6       That Membership of any Active member who fails to attend at least one Meeting during a period of two years shall lapse, unless the explanation given by such Member for non-attendance is considered satisfactory by the Committee.

7       That the CLUB be administered by a Committee consisting of the President, Past President, the Secretary, the Treasurer and four other members.

8       That the subscription be £40.00 per annum or such sum as may be decided from time to time by a General Meeting of the CLUB. The financial year of the CLUB shall commence on October 1st of each year.

9       That all monies received on behalf of the CLUB be paid into the CLUB account at the NatWest Bank, 40 Whitgift Centre, Croydon, CR0 1UJ. (Account number: 13413767. Sort code: 60-50-01.) The Treasurer to be mandated as sole signatory of the CLUB account including the option to use internet banking for transactions when appropriate.

# Traditions and Guidance

Membership.

When considering names to be invited to become a member, a criterion espoused by Alan Moule (former President and Archivist) "is he or she clubbable?" is important. The relaxed, friendly , social atmosphere of the Club is essential.

Honorary Membership.

On occasion this has been given to our overseas hosts as they almost invariably make a big effort on our behalf. It is a way of thanking them but it also keeps the name of the Club to the fore.

Relationships.

The Club is a forum where confidential matters can be discussed and know that such discussions always remain confidential.

Meetings.

At the Autumn Meeting, normally the subjects presented by the lecturers are on topics other than oral and maxillofacial surgery, There will be occasions when it is sensible to vary this pattern.

The Spring Meeting is normally abroad and is concerned with our specialty.

Annual General Meetings.

We try to be succinct as possible and try to avoid committeeism,

"Points of Order" are frowned upon! It is important that the incoming President is properly briefed on "current business".

The Dinner.

The tradition is at present that there are no formal speeches.

The President always gives the Loyal toast.

This then allows a senior member of the club to propose a vote of thanks to the President for arranging the Scientific Program and to thank the speakers.

There have been notable contributions in the past from members who have entertained the assembled company with their wit. This is not formal and is therefore allowable.

# Rupert Sutton Taylor - A brief Biography

Rupert Sutton Taylor was born in Carrig Byrne, County Wexford on July 18, 1905. He was educated at Newtown School Waterford. His professional training in Dentistry was at the Royal Dental Hospital of London qualifying LDS RCS England in 1928; his Medical training was at the Middlesex Hospital where he qualified LRCP MRCS in 1930. He was elected FDS RCS England in 1948.

Although an Irishman he spent his professional life in England specialising in oral surgery and was possibly the first man to limit his practice entirely to oral surgery. In 1928 he was commissioned into the Royal Army Medical Corp (Territorial Army) and was promoted major in 1938 and Lieutenant Colonel in 1942. During the 1939-45 war he was Commanding Officer 127 Light Field Ambulance and 146 Field Ambulance. He was decorated an Officer of the Order of the British Empire (Military Division) in 1945. He was the Commanding Officer 161 Field Ambulance (Territorial Army) 1957-58 and was made Honorary Colonel Medical Units 54 (East Anglia) Infantry Division 1959-1966. In 1959 he was appointed an Officer of the Order of St John and made Commander in 1961.

His civilian achievements were notable. After qualifying in dentistry in 1928 he became the dental house surgeon at the Middlesex hospital followed by the appointment of clinical assistant to the dental department at the Westminster Hospital, 1929-31. His rise to the Consultant ranks can only be described as meteoric: he was appointed to the Seamen's Hospital Greenwich in 1930 as Consultant, holding the appointment until his retirement in 1970.

During the early 1930s he held several clinical posts: at the Nose Ear and Throat Hospital, the National Hospital Queen Square and in 1937 he was appointed Consultant at the Westminster Hospital. When the link between the Westminster Hospital and Queen Mary's Hospital Roehampton occurred in 1962 he was Senior Consultant in oral surgery and held the appointment until his retirement. He was made Honorary Consultant to both the Westminster Hospital teaching group and the Seamen's Hospital in 1970. He was an examiner in dental surgery and materia medica at Queens University Belfast both before and after the war.

He served on the Representative Board of the British Dental Association for many years, where his great contribution had been in the field

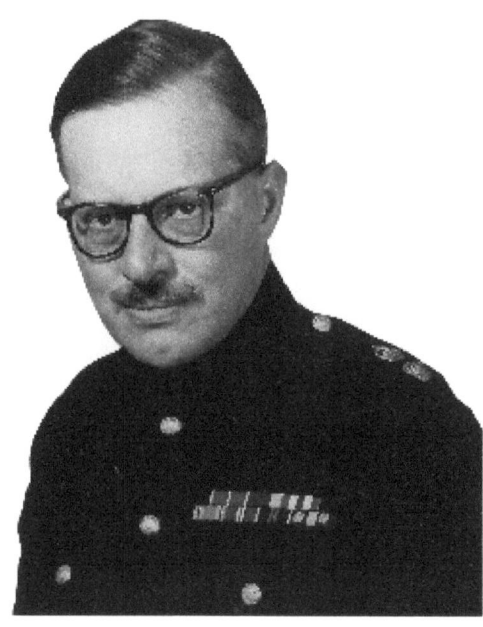

of hospital dentistry. It could be said he was one of the architects of it. A past President of the Hospitals Group he had the distinction of being the first chairman of the Central Dental Consultants and Specialists Committee, now the Central Committee for Hospital Dental Services. As well as this, he had also served for several years as the chairman of the London Executive Council (NHS).

Apart from giving birth to the Oral Surgery Club and becoming the first secretary and treasurer from 1937 to 1962, when he became the president, he was a member of the steering committee of the now British Association of Oral and Maxillofacial Surgeons, formerly the British Association of Oral Surgeons. He was a member of the inaugural Council in 1962 and president in 1965. In 1966 he became president of the Odontological Section of the Royal Society of Medicine. In 1969 Rupert Sutton Taylor was made a fellow of the British Dental Association which was a great honour and recognition of the great contribution that he had made to dentistry.

But what of the man? Above all he was a gentleman, irascible at times with a fiery temperament. However any altercations were quickly forgotten and underneath it all was a man of great kindness who fully supported all his staff: trainees, nurses, technicians and secretaries alike. There are many consultants and some professors who followed Sutton Taylor and had much to be thankful for the help and guidance he had given them in their careers.

Rupert Sutton Taylor had great administrative ability. Among the many successes was his successful attempt at getting the necessary finance to build the new Department of oral and maxillofacial surgery at Queen Mary's Hospital Roehampton. In those days it was a huge sum of money and in recognition of his feat the Minister of Health himself came and cut the first sod for the foundations and kept the spade to remind him of the occasion.

He spent his retirement in the Isle of Man concerned with his early interest in the growing of exotic plants and shrubs. A memorable 80th birthday celebration was held in his honour at the Royal College of Surgeons. He died at Ramsay on the Isle of Man on February April 4, 1986.

# Images

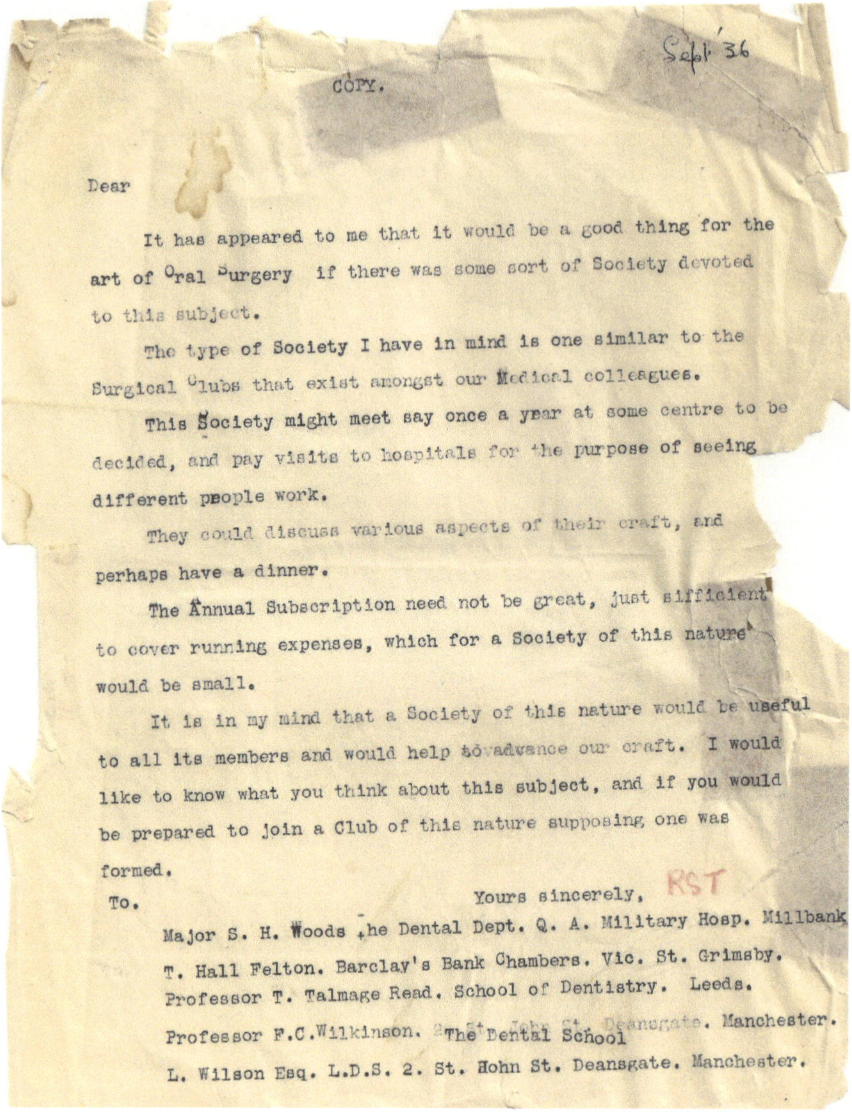

Sept '36

COPY.

Dear

It has appeared to me that it would be a good thing for the art of Oral Surgery if there was some sort of Society devoted to this subject.

The type of Society I have in mind is one similar to the Surgical Clubs that exist amongst our Medical colleagues.

This Society might meet say once a year at some centre to be decided, and pay visits to hospitals for the purpose of seeing different people work.

They could discuss various aspects of their craft, and perhaps have a dinner.

The Annual Subscription need not be great, just sifficient to cover running expenses, which for a Society of this nature would be small.

It is in my mind that a Society of this nature would be useful to all its members and would help to advance our craft. I would like to know what you think about this subject, and if you would be prepared to join a Club of this nature supposing one was formed.

Yours sincerely,

RST

To.

Major S. H. Woods The Dental Dept. Q. A. Military Hosp. Millbank

T. Hall Felton. Barclay's Bank Chambers. Vic. St. Grimsby.

Professor T. Talmage Read. School of Dentistry. Leeds.

Professor F.C.Wilkinson. The Dental School Manchester.

L. Wilson Esq. L.D.S. 2. St. Hohn St. Deansgate. Manchester.

***Figure 1. Sutton Taylor's letter of 1936.***

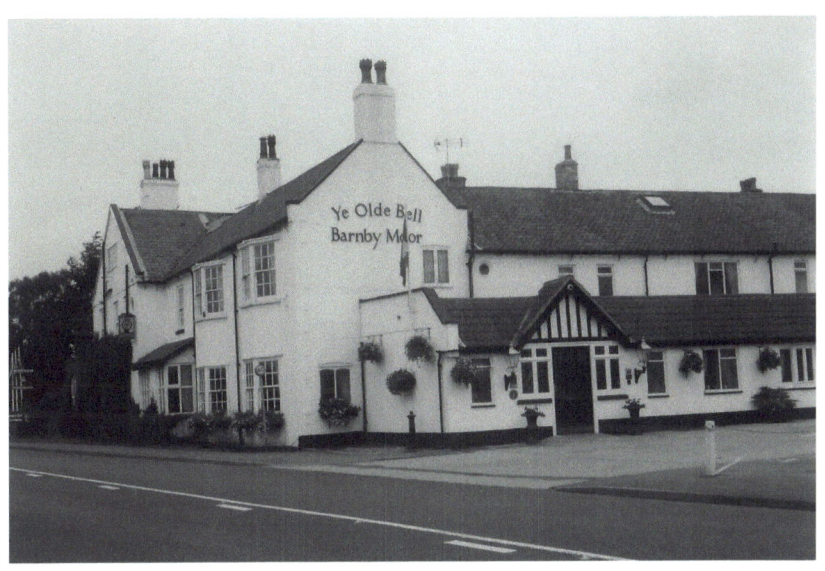

*Figure 2.* **Ye Old Bell Hotel, Barnby Moor.**

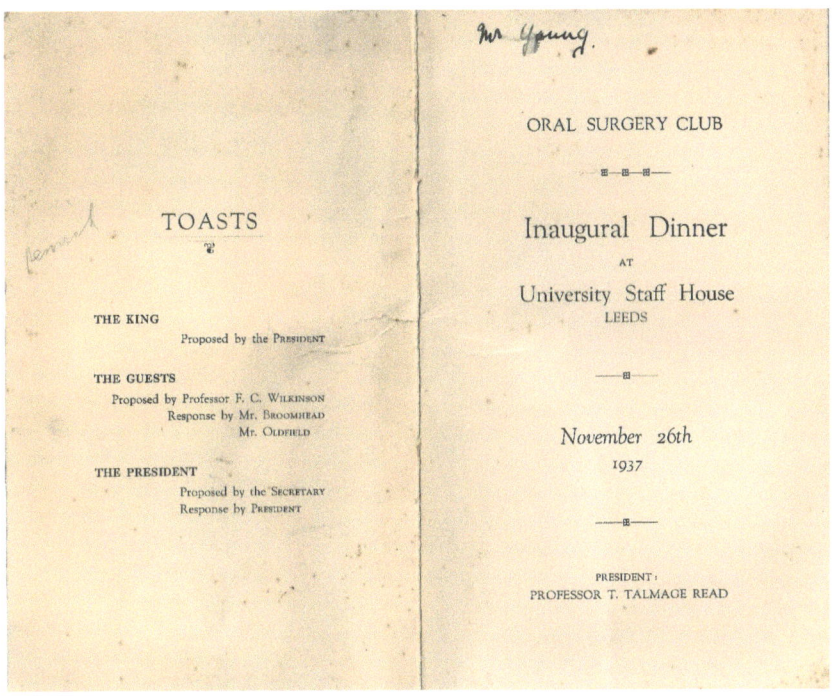

*Mr Young.*

ORAL SURGERY CLUB

Inaugural Dinner
AT
University Staff House
LEEDS

November 26th
1937

PRESIDENT:
PROFESSOR T. TALMAGE READ

TOASTS

THE KING
    Proposed by the PRESIDENT

THE GUESTS
    Proposed by Professor F. C. WILKINSON
        Response by Mr. BROOMHEAD
            Mr. OLDFIELD

THE PRESIDENT
    Proposed by the SECRETARY
    Response by PRESIDENT

*Figure 3.* **The Inaugural Dinner**

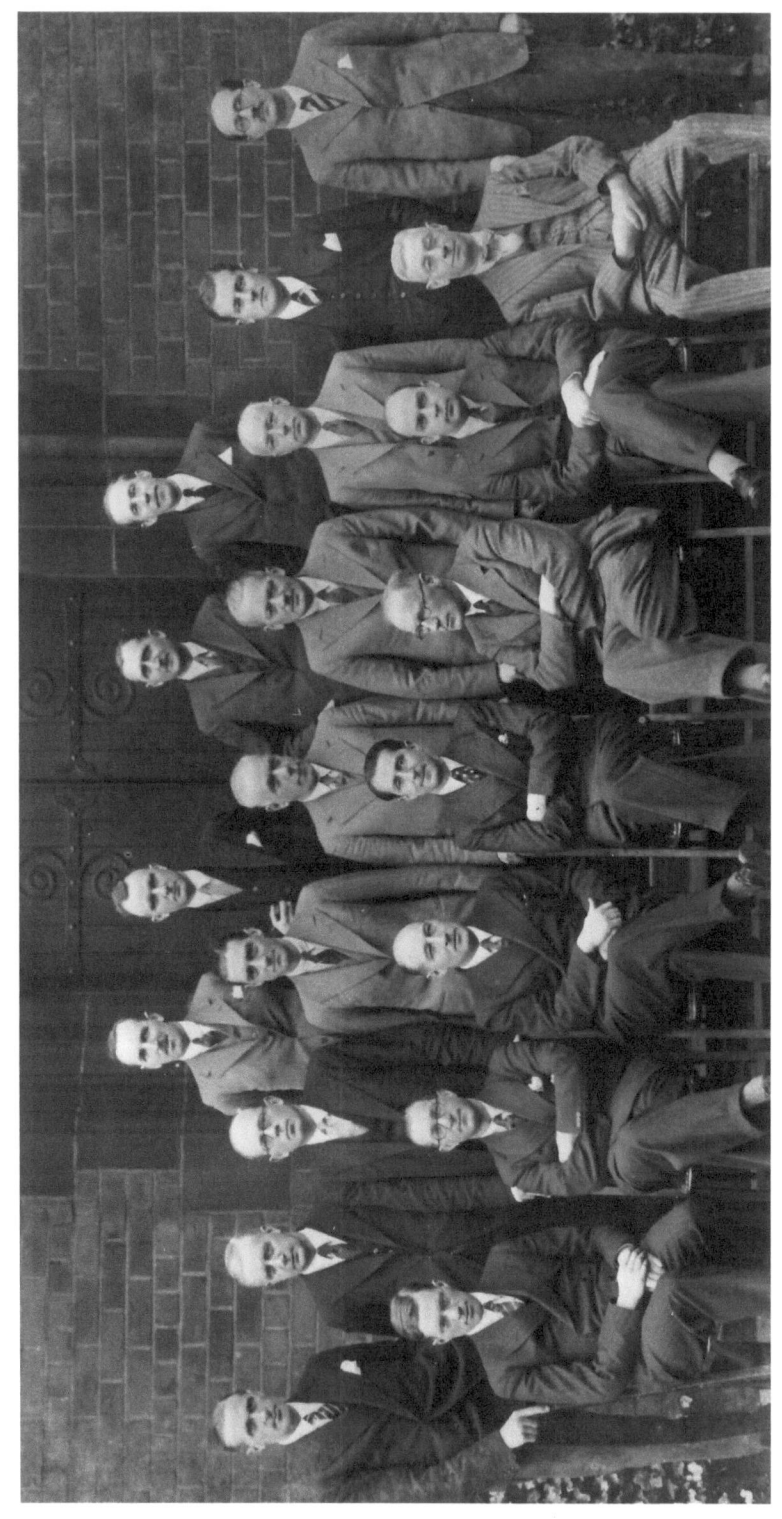

**The first club meeting  Leeds. 26th November 1937** *Back row: L MacLaren Young, Maj. A Drummond, AM Milne, A Cubie. **Middle row:** JSH Collinge, T Jackson, R Payne, LR Marsh, D Fyfe, A Pain, S Hanreck, JD Cambrooke, C Read. **Front row:** RS Taylor, Maj. SH Woods, Prof. FC Wilkinson, Prof. Talmage Read, AE Rowlett, T Hall Felton, AM Nodine*

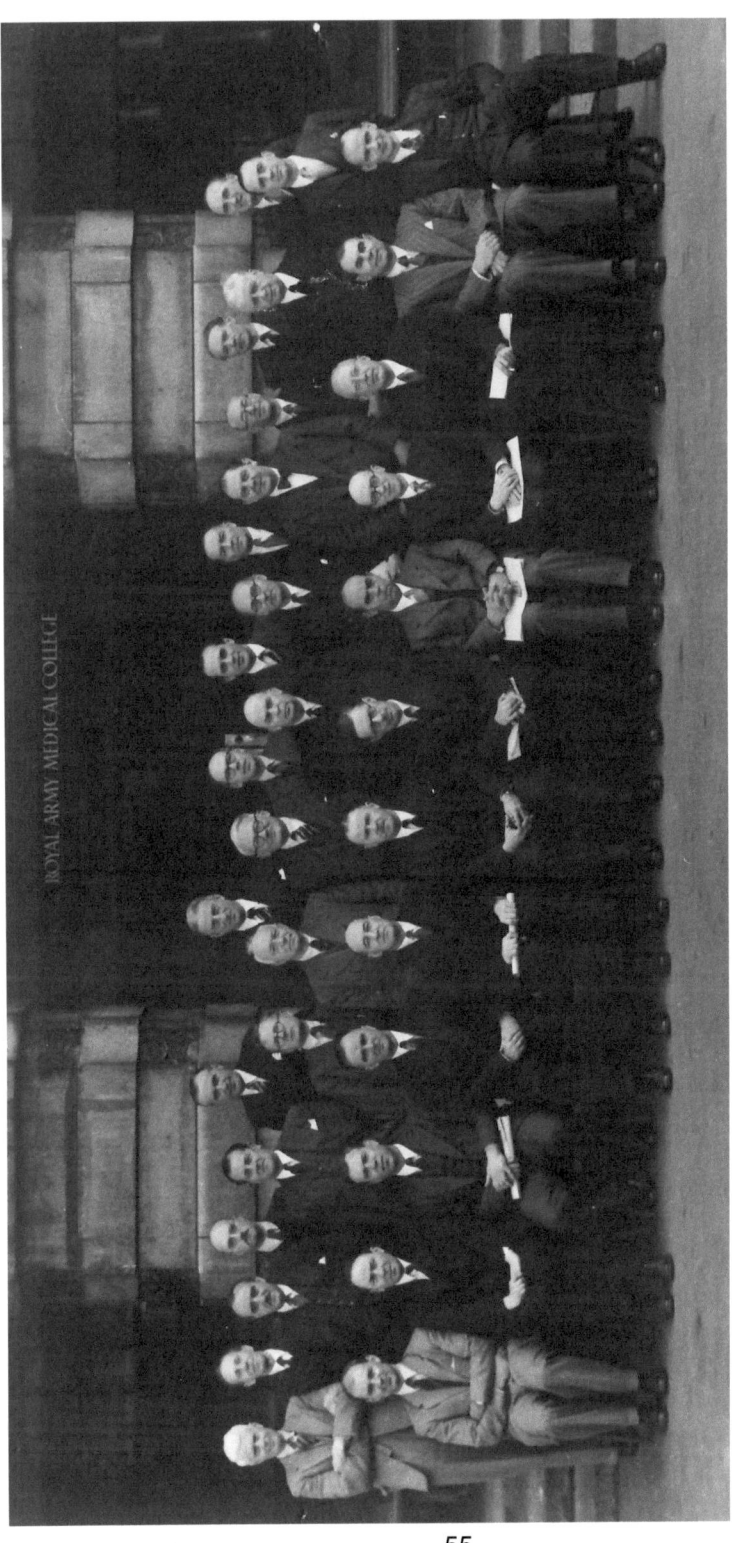

*Meeting, 28th October 1950 Royal Army College Millbank London*
**Back Row:** (Duckworth RAMC) Cubie Collinge Vidler Moule Steadman McPhee ?RAMC Selby-Brown. **Middle Row:** (Hargreaves RAMC) Janes Cambrook FitzGibbon Hanreck Pain Felton Farris Hardy Woods Jackson ?RAMC **Front Row:** Benson Boyes Darling Drummond Wilkinson (RAMC) Taylor Gibb Stones ?RAMC ?RAMC Ward

55

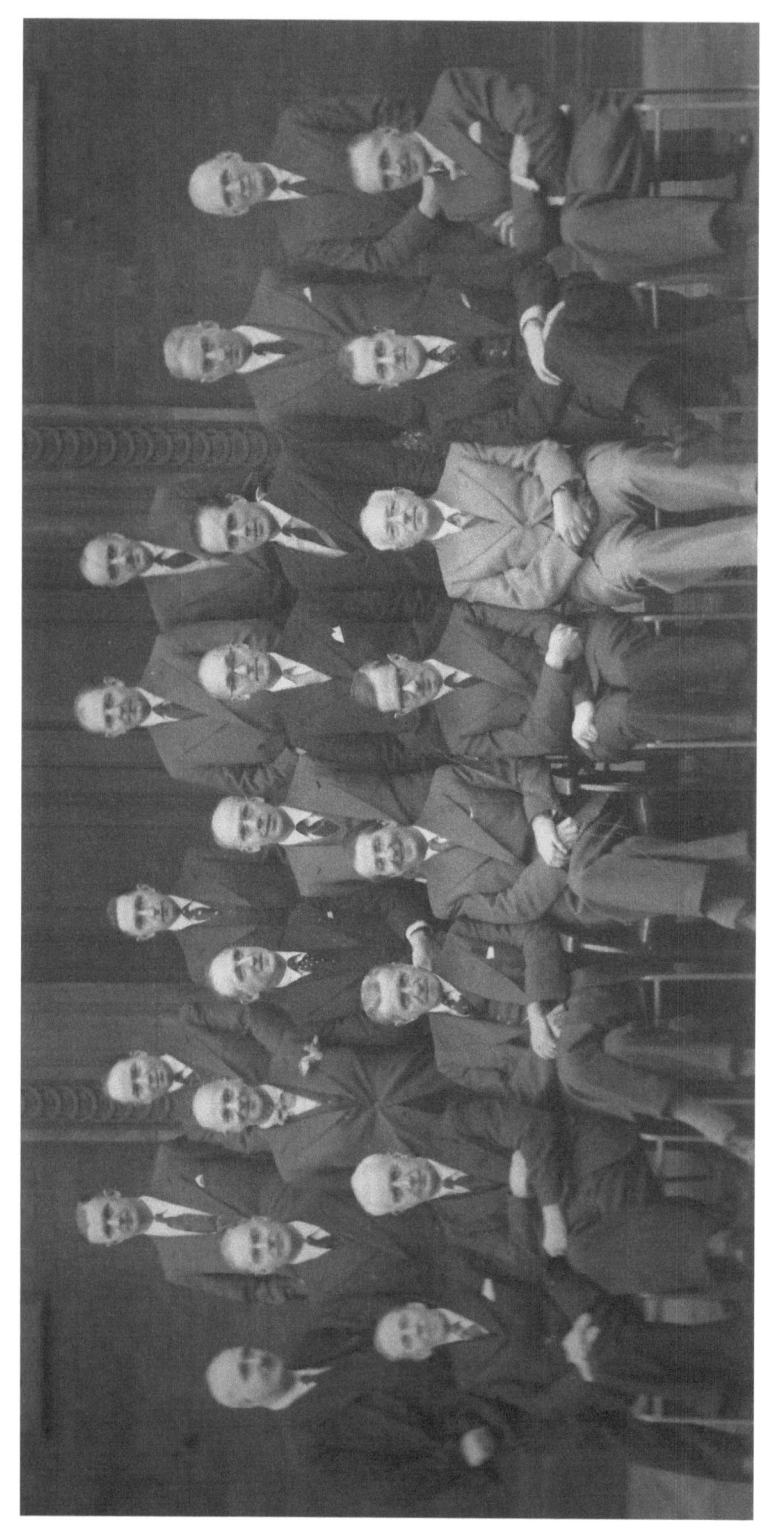

*Meeting 18th December 1953   Leeds Dental School.*
***Back Row:*** *Monks   Boyes Snawdon Hardy Janes **Middle Row:** Middleton Fickling Scott Selby-Brown Moule Farris Steadman   Vidler Meeson **Front Row:***   *Cubie Jackson Broderick Talmage Read Taylor Hanreck Cambrook Collinge*

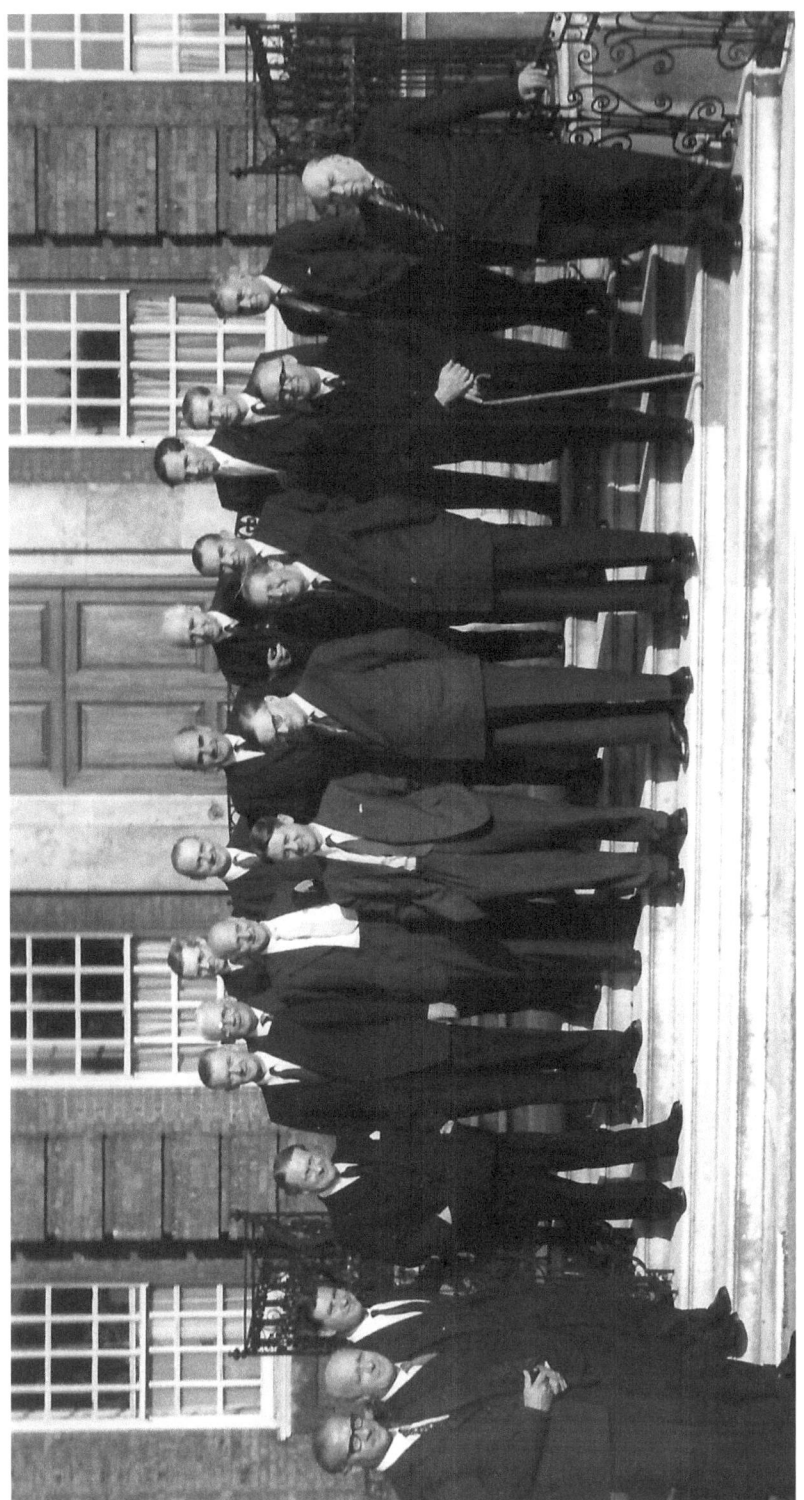

*Meeting  Roehampton 1963*

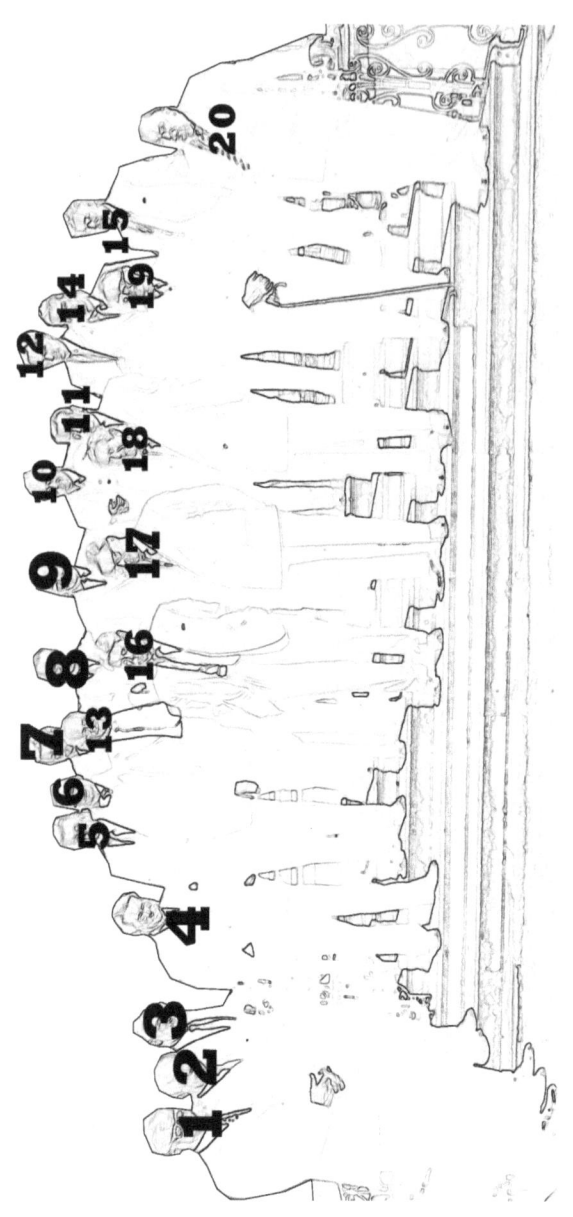

1 Ireland
2 Craddock Henry
3 Whitlock
4 Rowe
5 Monks
6 Pain
7 Cook
8 Maclennon
9 Warrack
10 Middleton
11 Walker
12 Bramley
13 Scott
14 Heslop
15 Hogan
16 Howe
17 Taylor (President)
18 Talmage Read
19 Fitzgibbon
20 Felton

58

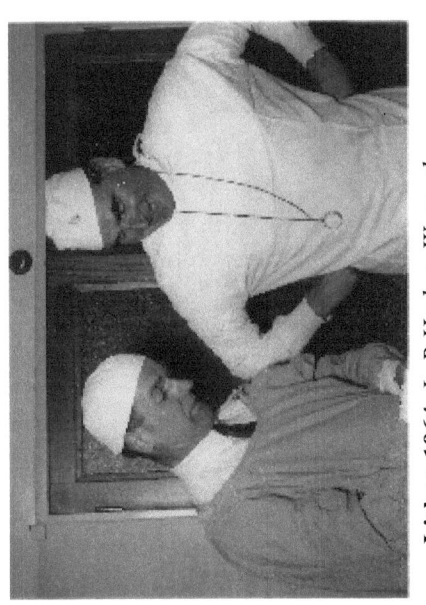

**Lisbon 1964** *L–R Heslop, Warrack*

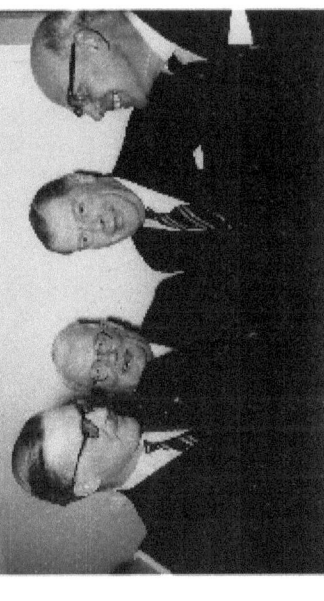

**Lisbon 1964** *L - R S Taylor, Pain, D V Taylor, Moule*

**Lisbon 1964** *L-R Warrack, Staff, Howe, Heslop, Taylor*

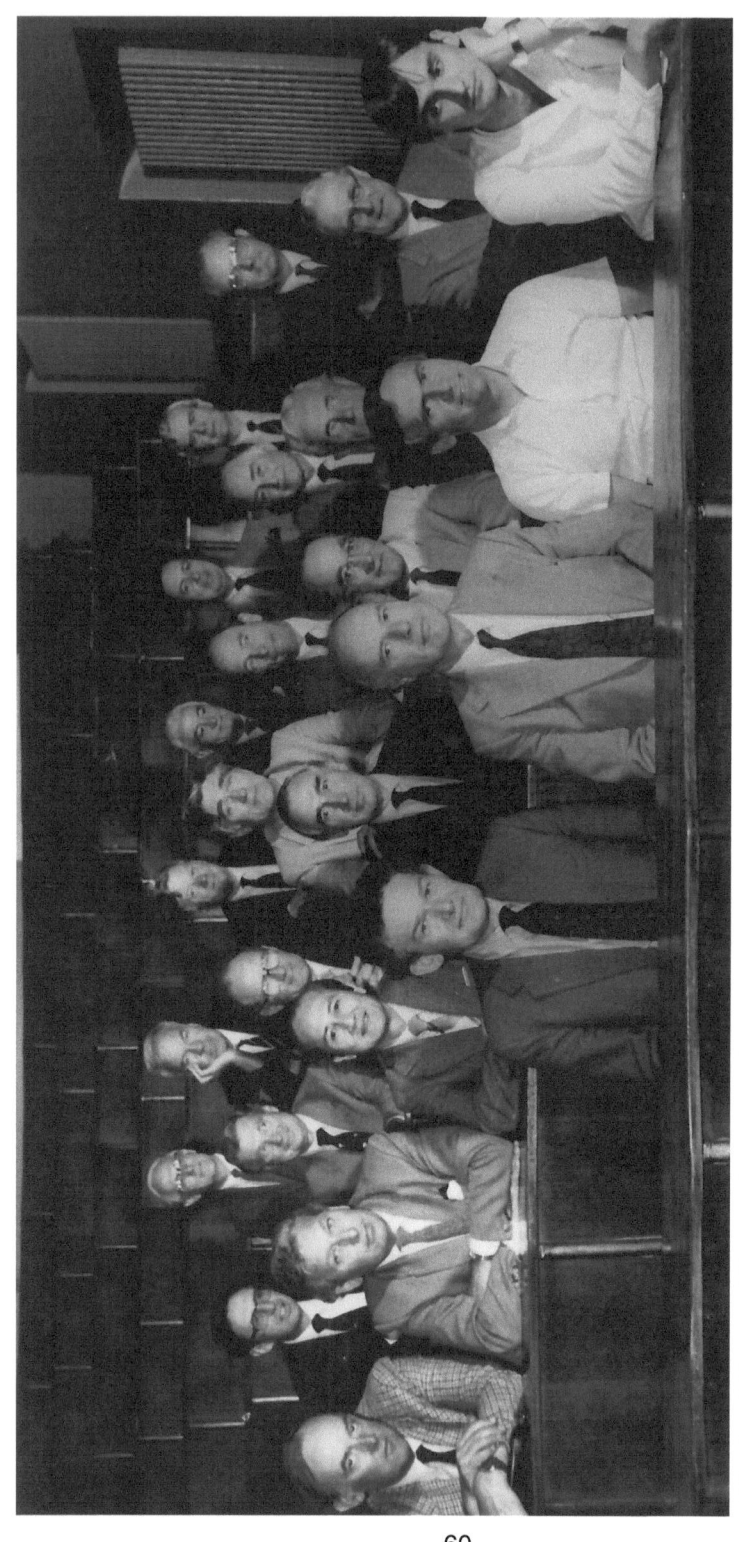

*Meeting 11th June 1985* **Budapest** Professor Georgi Szabo
**4th Row:** Gibson Jones Smith Downton Cheney O'Neill **3rd Row:** B Morgan Whitlock Emerson Mason Penney Clarke McGowan **2nd row:** Banks Manning (visitor) Ray Selwyn Merkx Cook **Front Row:** Bradley Alty Szabo Staff Member

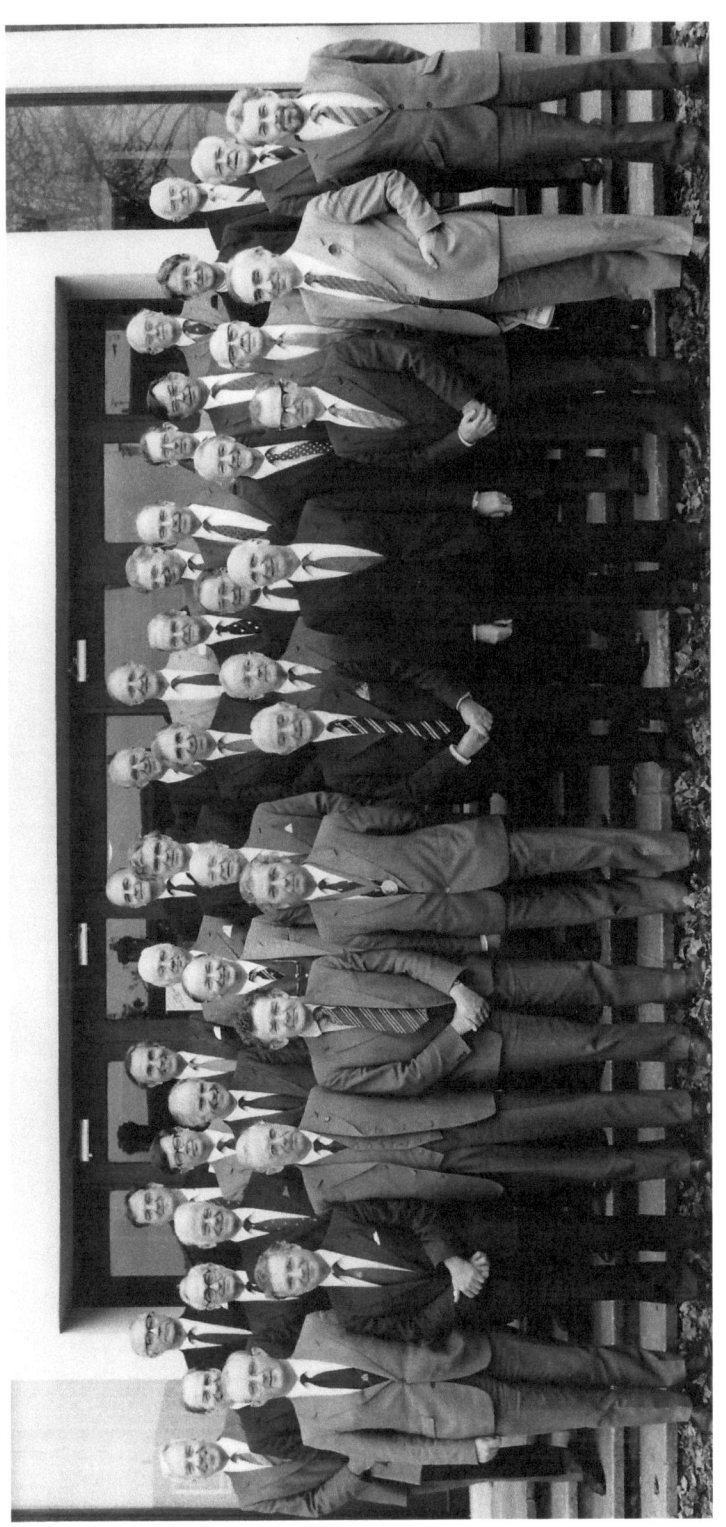

*Meeting 31ˢᵗ October 1986 Stoke-on-Trent*

**4ᵗʰ Row:** *E Morgan Quant Bramley Rayne James Hardman Smith Newell Gibson* **3ʳᵈ Row:** *Jones Crewe Hall MacLennan Mason Simpson Heslop Penney Wilson Howe Fickling* **2ⁿᵈ Row:** *Williams Poswillo Alty Henderson Henry Lewars Selwyn Awty Moule Hogan* **Front Row:** *McGowan Whitlock Cook J Bradley Manning Downton Hamilton Gray Ray P Bradley*

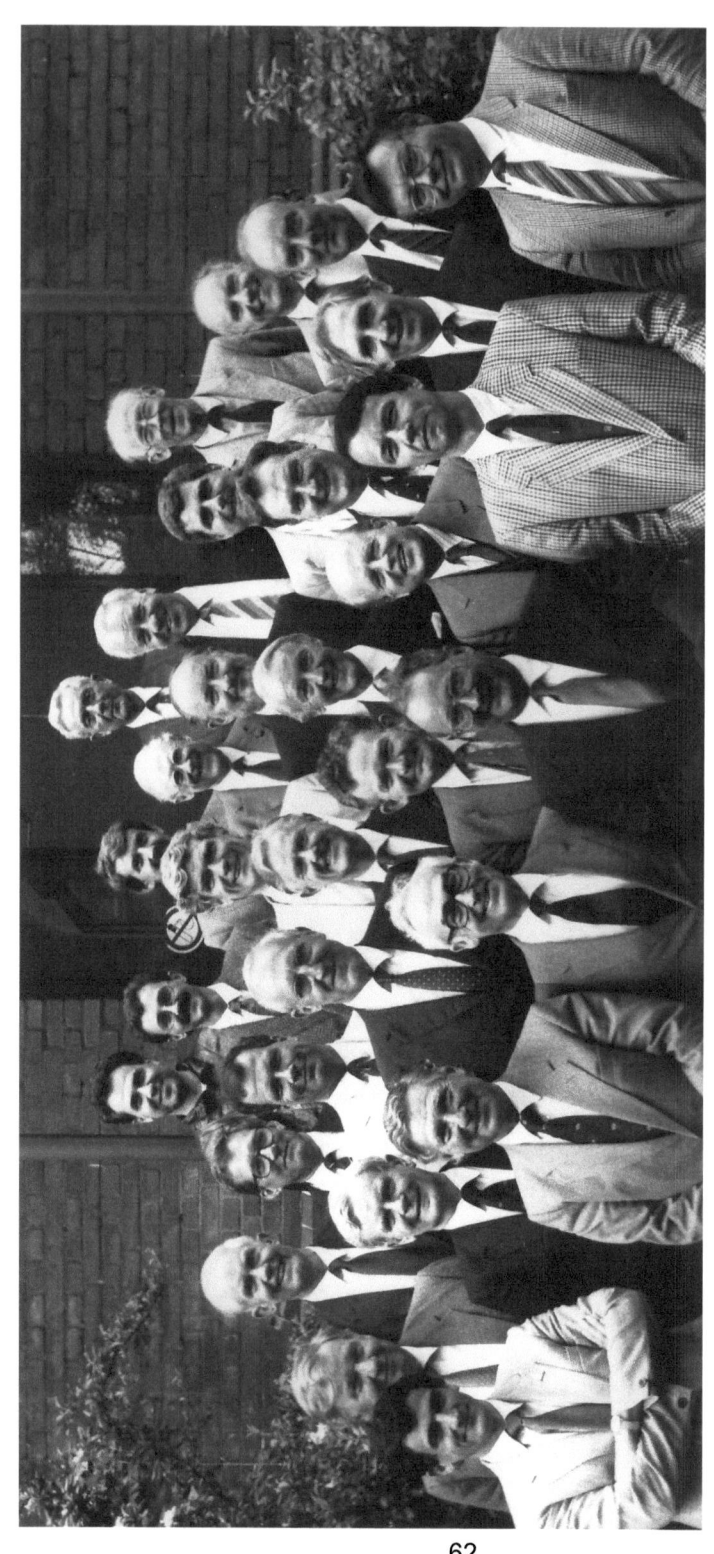

*Meeting June 1988  Cologne  Professor Hans-Dieter Pape*

**5th Row:** *(staff)  (staff)  (staff)  Cook  Merkx  Jones  English* **4th Row:** *Sear  Rowse  Mason  Henderson  McAndrew  Alty* **3rd Row:** *Barnard  Gorman  Awty  Quant  Banks* **2nd Row:** *Smith  O'Neil  James  Bradley  Pape  Simpson* **Front Row:** *Ward  Booth  Whitlock  Crewe  Selwyn (staff)  Wilson*

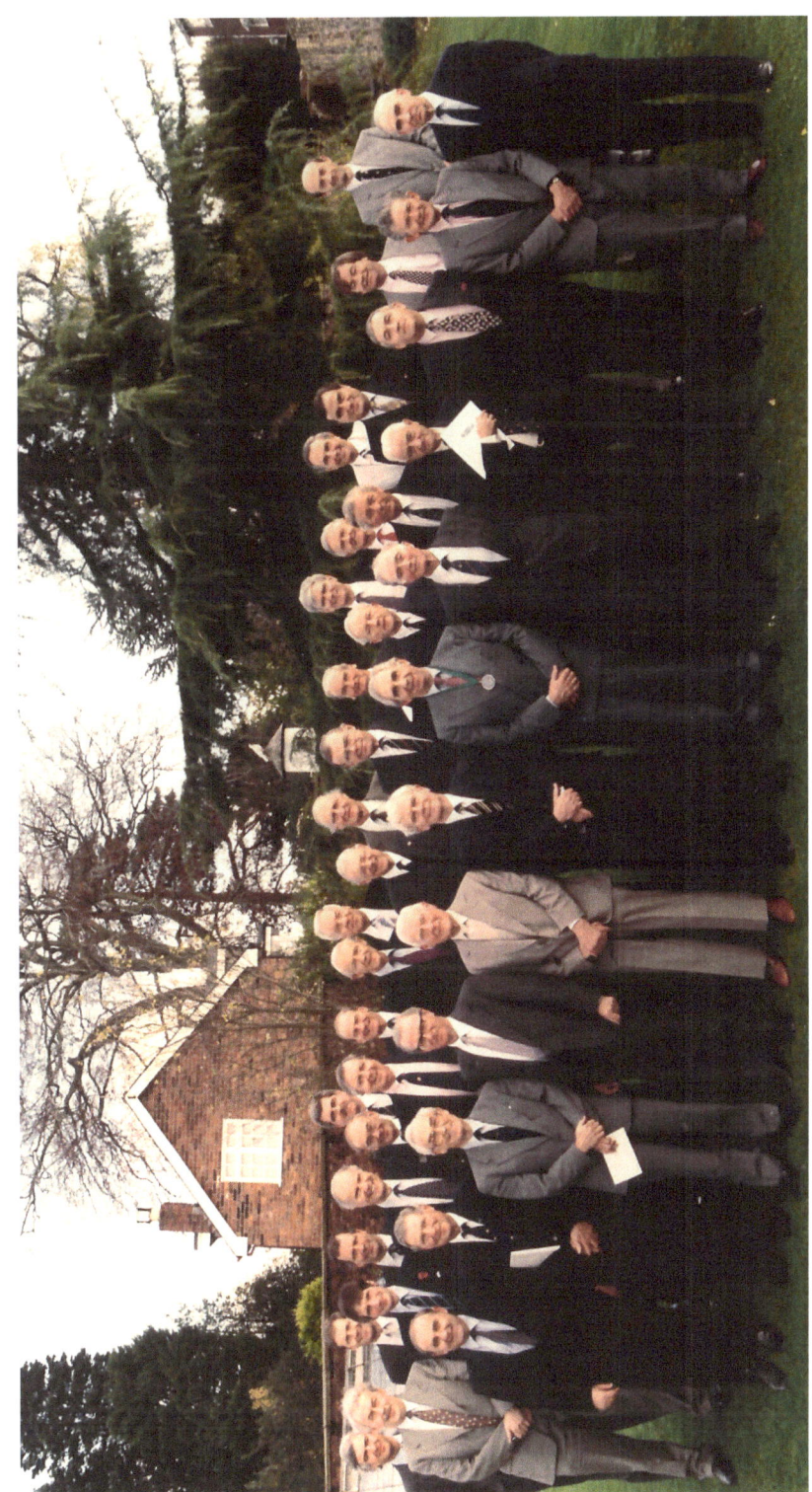

*Meeting November 1993 Alderley Edge*

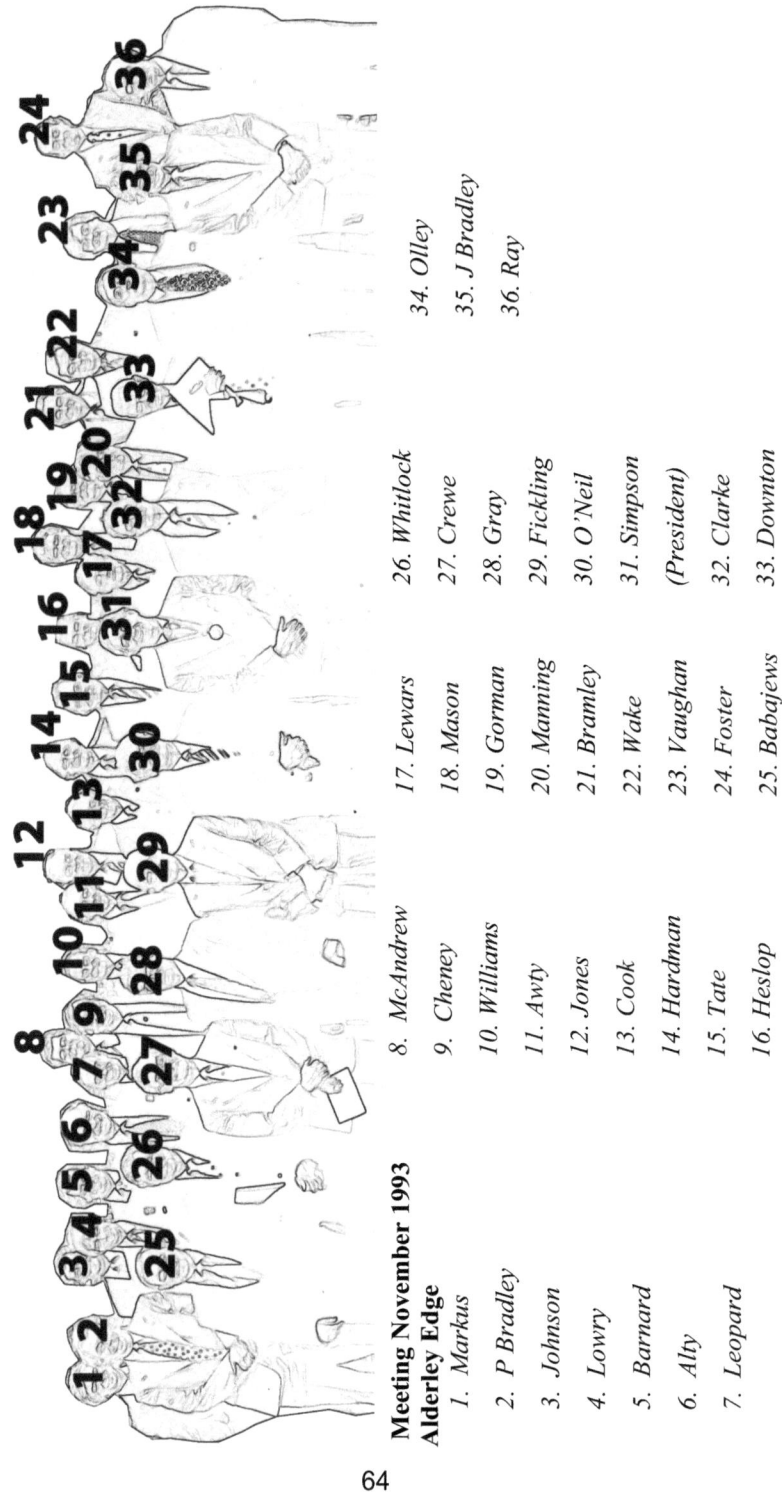

**Meeting November 1993**
**Alderley Edge**

1. Markus
2. P Bradley
3. Johnson
4. Lowry
5. Barnard
6. Alty
7. Leopard
8. McAndrew
9. Cheney
10. Williams
11. Awty
12. Jones
13. Cook
14. Hardman
15. Tate
16. Heslop
17. Lewars
18. Mason
19. Gorman
20. Manning
21. Bramley
22. Wake
23. Vaughan
24. Foster
25. Babajews
26. Whitlock
27. Crewe
28. Gray
29. Fickling
30. O'Neil
31. Simpson
    (President)
32. Clarke
33. Downton
34. Olley
35. J Bradley
36. Ray

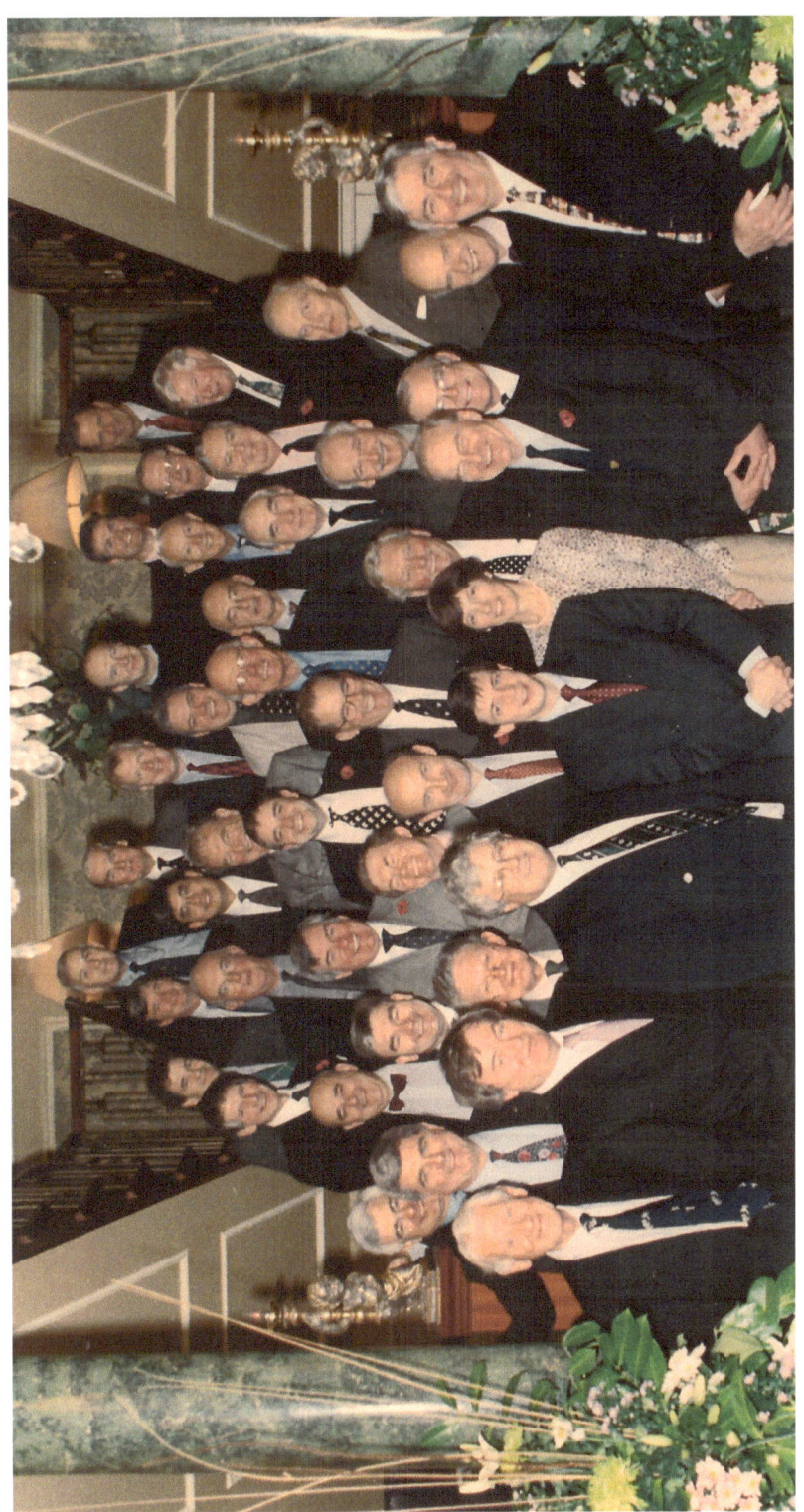

Meeting November 2001 Macclesfield

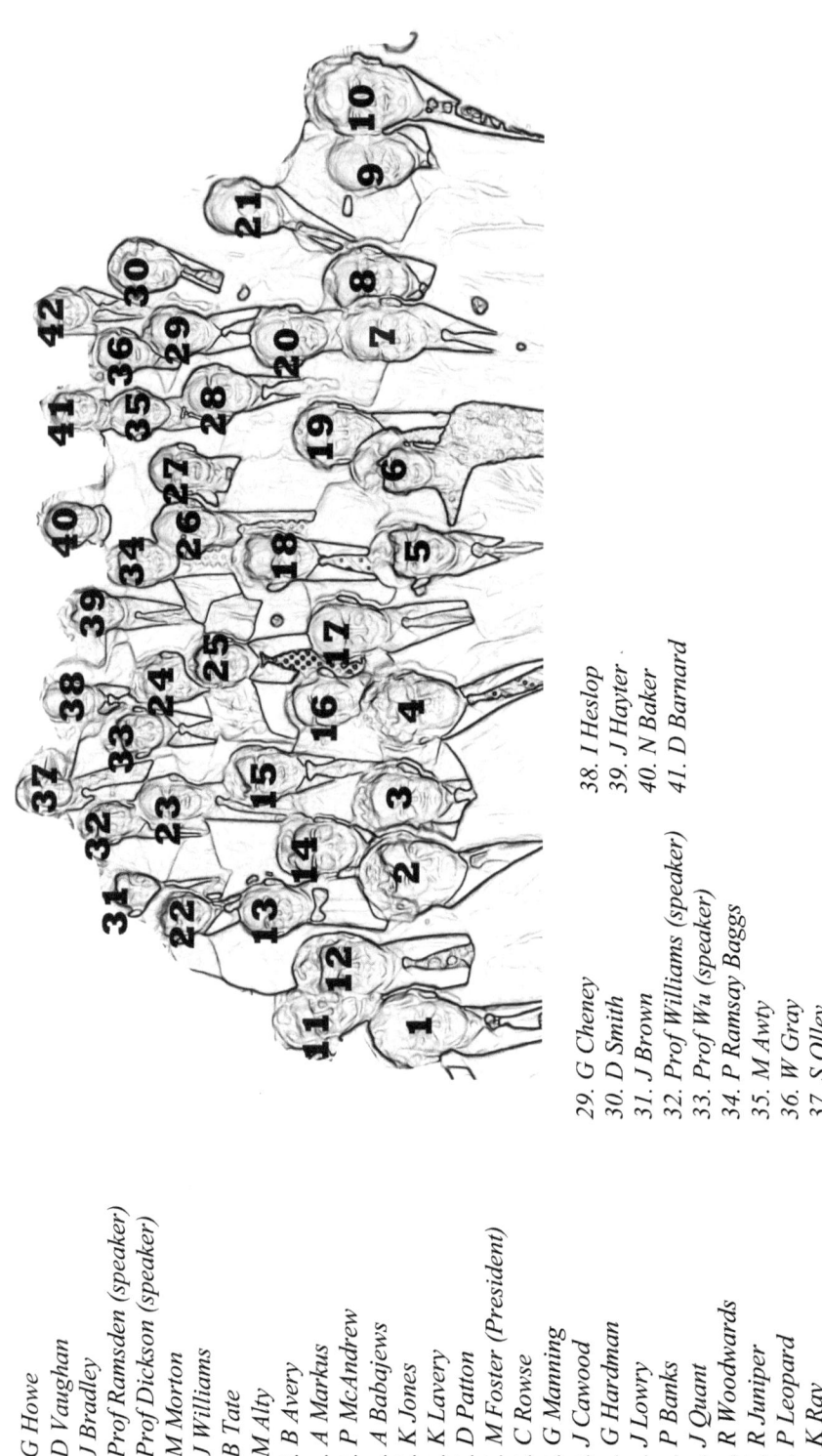

1 G Howe
2. D Vaughan
3. J Bradley
4. Prof Ramsden (speaker)
5. Prof Dickson (speaker)
6. M Morton
7. J Williams
8. B Tate
9. M Alty
10. B Avery
11. A Markus
12. P McAndrew
13. A Babajews
14. K Jones
15. K Lavery
16. D Patton
17. M Foster (President)
18. C Rowse
19. G Manning
20. J Cawood
21. G Hardman
22. J Lowry
23. P Banks
24. J Quant
25. R Woodwards
26. R Juniper
27. P Leopard
28. K Ray
29. G Cheney
30. D Smith
31. J Brown
32. Prof Williams (speaker)
33. Prof Wu (speaker)
34. P Ramsay Baggs
35. M Awty
36. W Gray
37. S Olley
38. I Heslop
39. J Hayter
40. N Baker
41. D Barnard

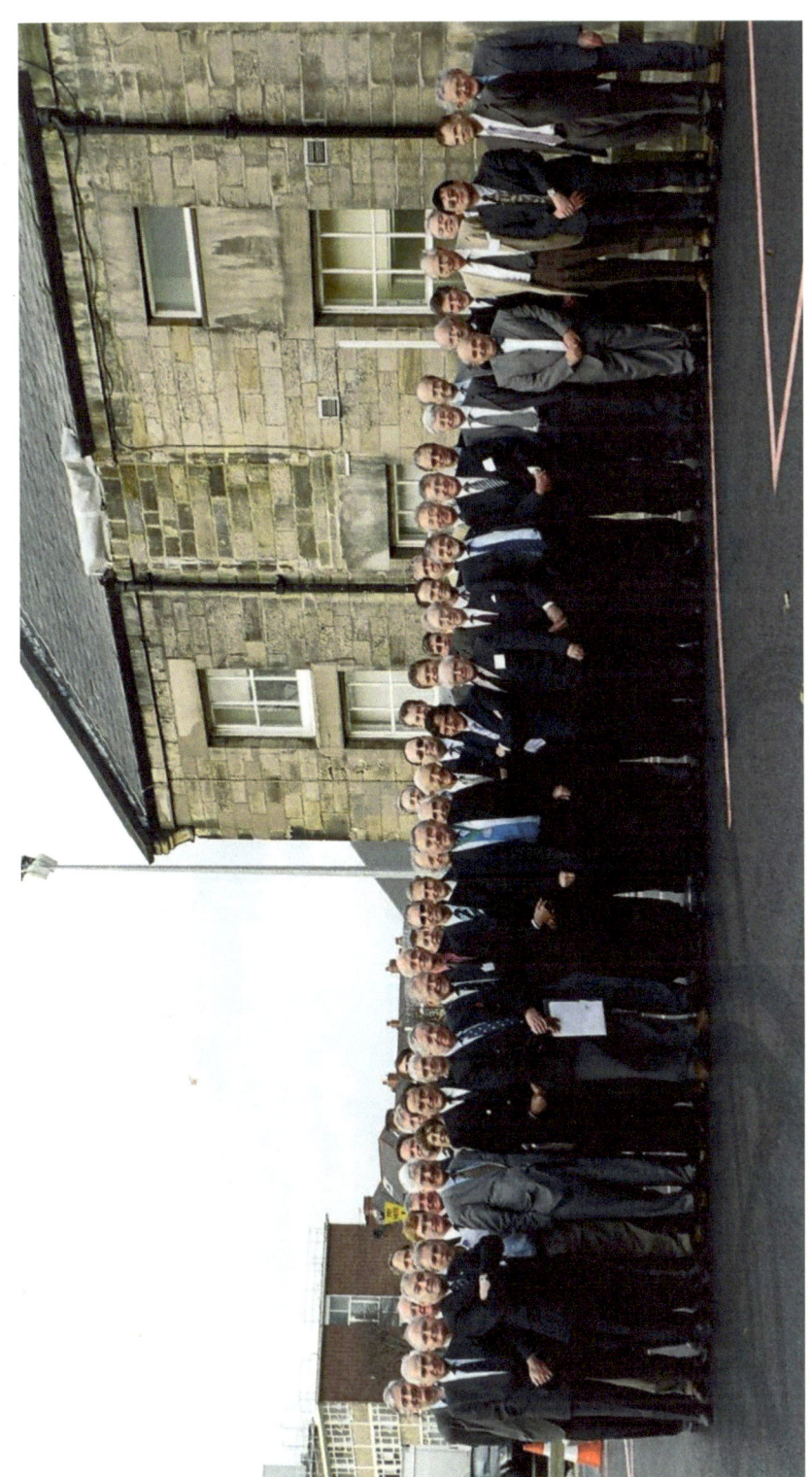

Meeting Newcastle 2006

1. Avery
2. Ray
3. Weller
4. McGowan
5. Olley
6. Simpson M
7. Macpherson
8. Boyd
9. Lavery
10. Markaus
11. McVicar
12. Morton
13. Hayter
14. Wake
15. Herold
16. Sadler
17. Cheney
18. Tate
19. Juniper
20. Renny
21. Bailey
22. Bramley
23. Penfold
24. J Hawkesford (president)
25. Simpson B
26. Frame
27. Awty
28. Sugar
29. Dover
30. Ward Booth
31. Smart
32. Adlam
33. Koppel
34. Newall
35. Lyons
36. Kreush
37. Woodwards
38. Hamlyn
39. Kendrick
40. Barnard
41. Lello
42. Foster
43. Babajews
44. Henderson
45. Lowry
46. Oldham
47. Ramsay Baggs
48. Ed Ong (Newcastle Lecturer)
49. Smyth
50. Bradley

68

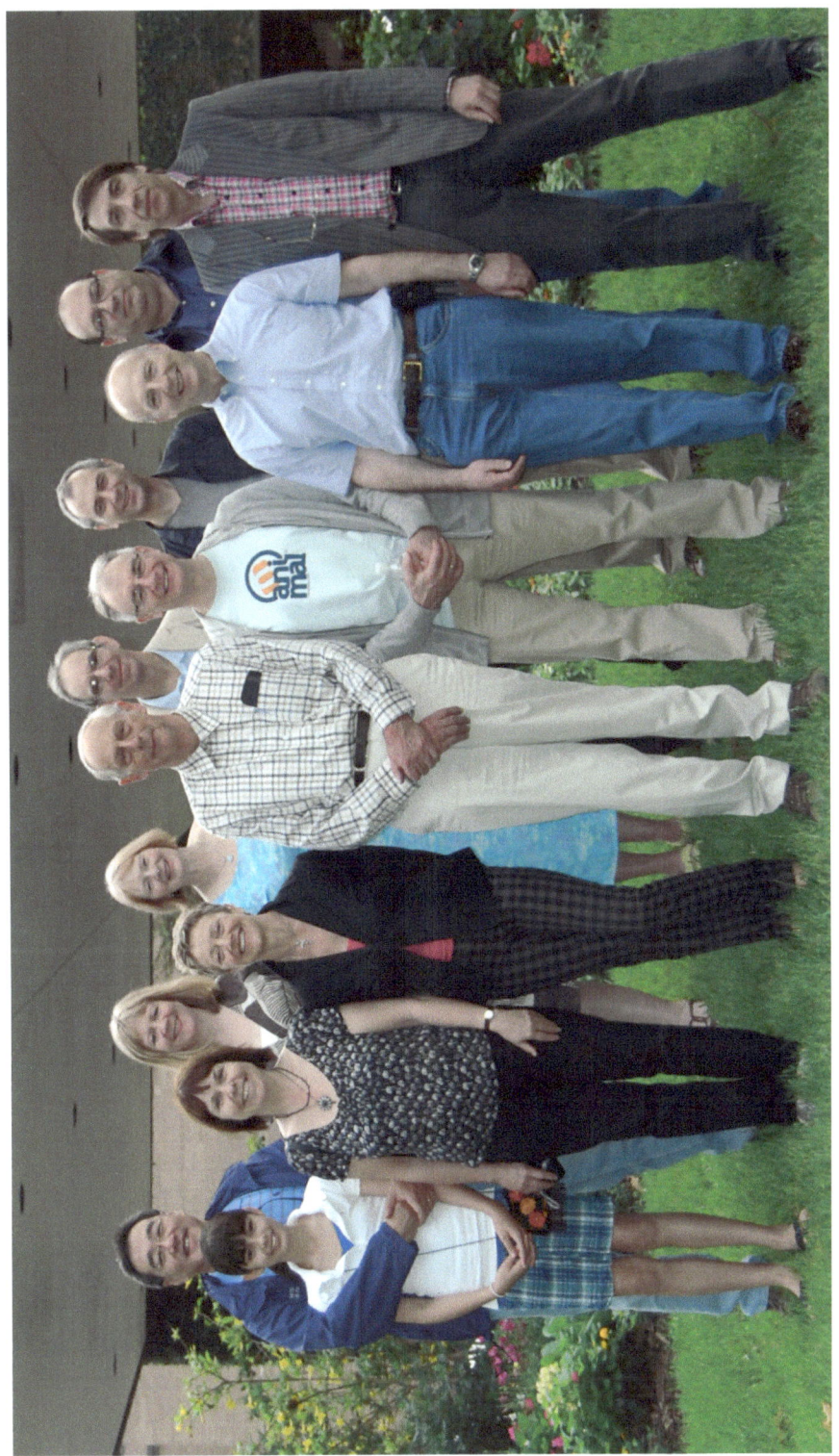

**Houston May 2009**

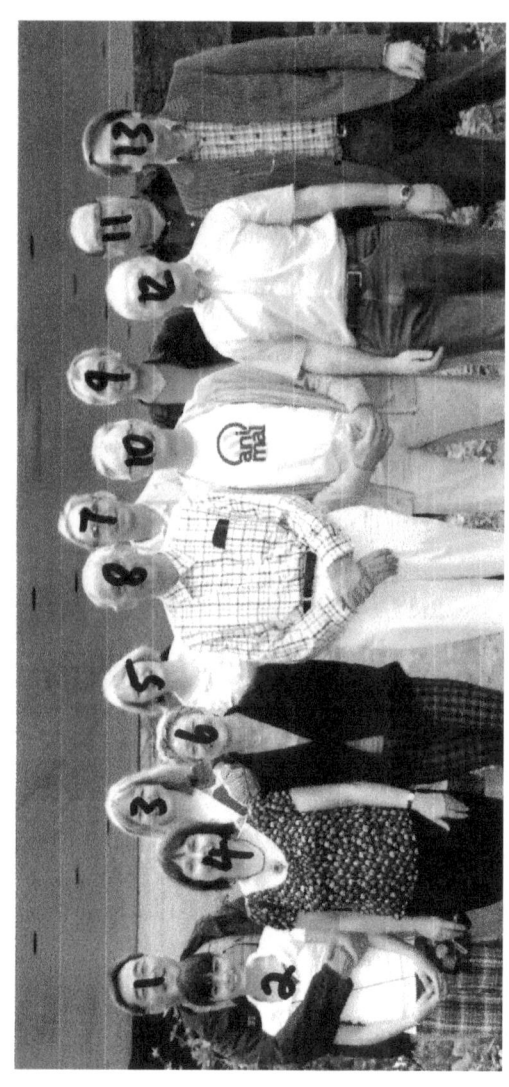

**Houston May 2009**

1. Mark Wong (host)
2. Lindsay Wong
3. Sheila Hislop
4. Maralyn Sadler
5. Chrsitine Bailey
6. Lindsay Wood
7. Malcolm Bailey
8. Lawrence Oldham
9. Stuart Hislop
10. Phillip Earl
11. Adrian Sugar
12. Graham Wood
13. Andrew Sadler

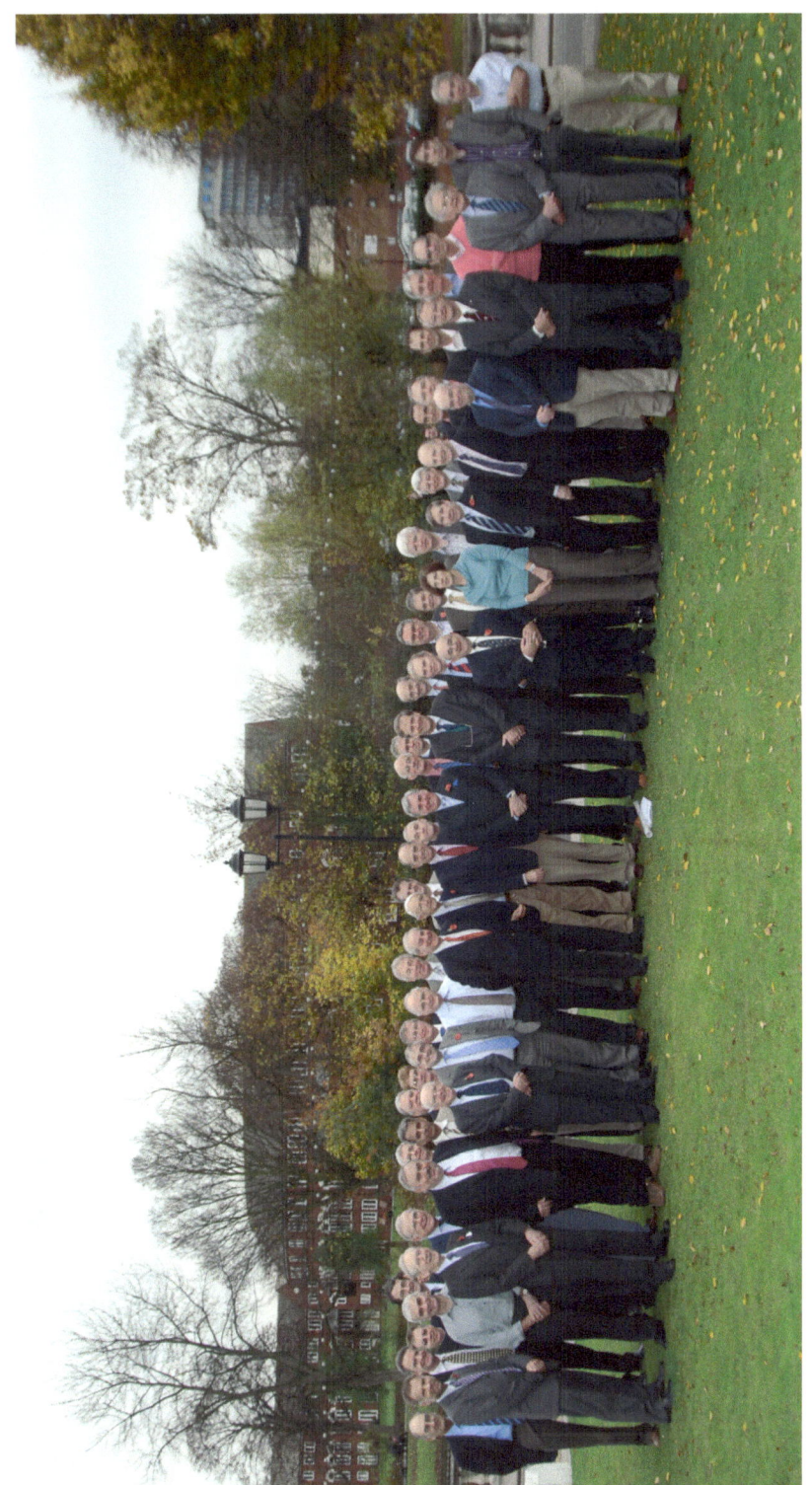

**Meeting Bedford 2009**

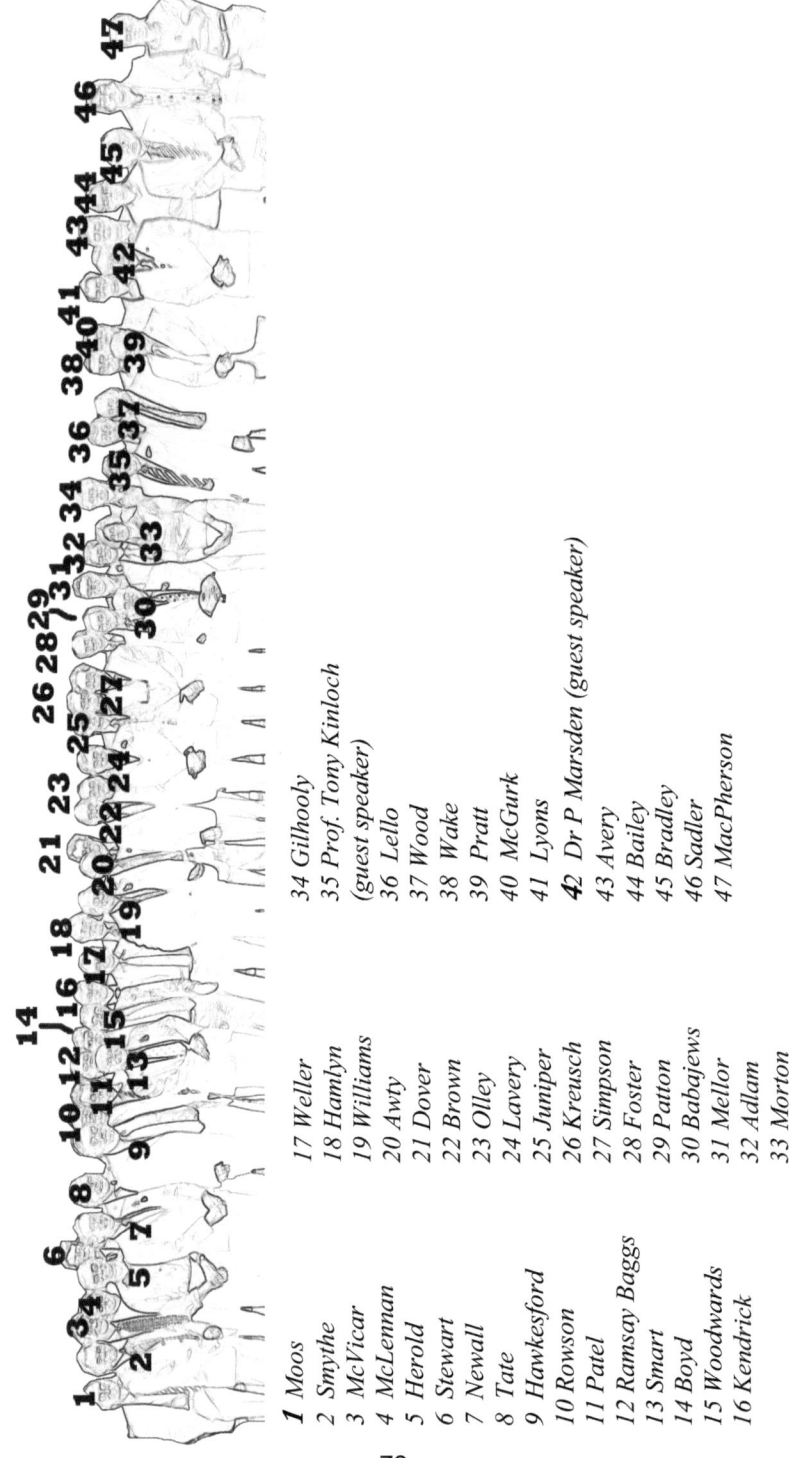

1 Moos
2 Smythe
3 McVicar
4 McLennan
5 Herold
6 Stewart
7 Newall
8 Tate
9 Hawkesford
10 Rowson
11 Patel
12 Ramsay Baggs
13 Smart
14 Boyd
15 Woodwards
16 Kendrick
17 Weller
18 Hamlyn
19 Williams
20 Awty
21 Dover
22 Brown
23 Olley
24 Lavery
25 Juniper
26 Kreusch
27 Simpson
28 Foster
29 Patton
30 Babajews
31 Mellor
32 Adlam
33 Morton
34 Gilhooly
35 Prof. Tony Kinloch
(guest speaker)
36 Lello
37 Wood
38 Wake
39 Pratt
40 McGurk
41 Lyons
42 Dr P Marsden (guest speaker)
43 Avery
44 Bailey
45 Bradley
46 Sadler
47 MacPherson

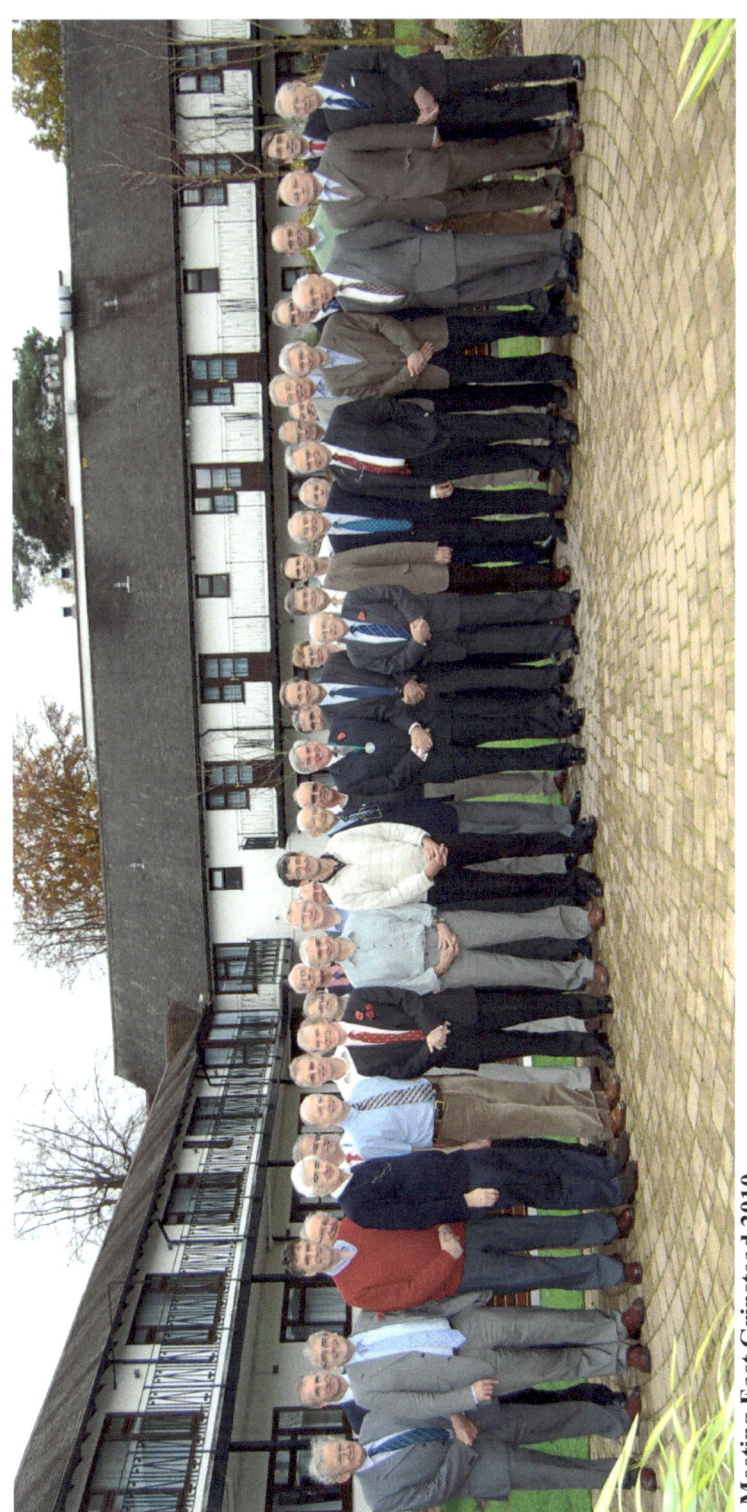

**Meeting East Grinstead 2010**

*L - R  Bradley Downie Woodwards Martin Penfold Markus Newman  Wood Fardy Patten Davidson Juniper Herold Hayter  Earl Stewart Awry Banks President Ken Lavery Webster  Simpson Boyd Smart Adlam Lyons Williams MacPherson  Ramsay-Baggs Barnard Hawkesford Hamlyn Rowson Bailey Cawood Brown Weller Sadler Newall*

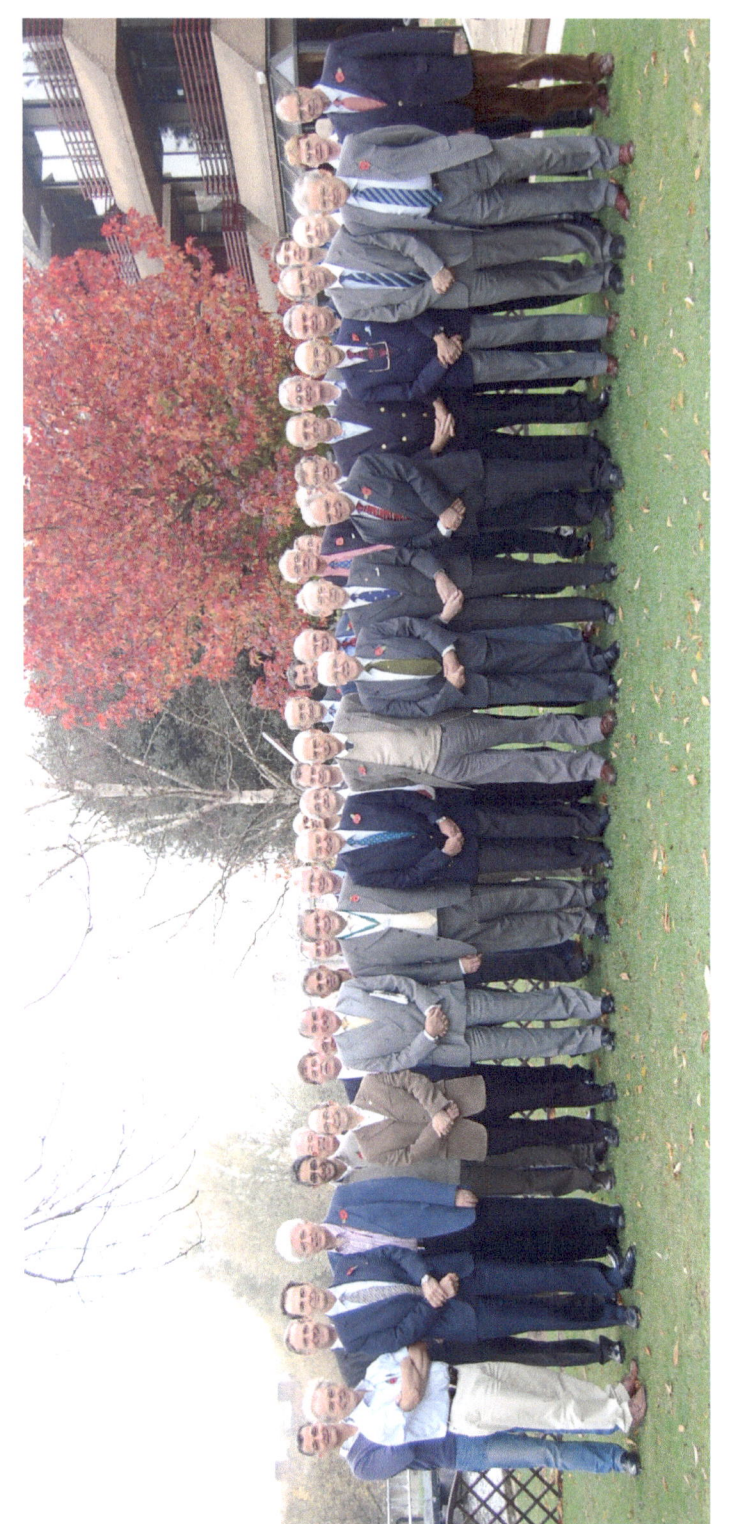

**Cambridge 10-11th November 2011**
**L - R** *Camilleri MacPherson Simpson Lyons Gilhooly Visavadia Hamlyn Evans Rennie Lavery Patel Hislop Adlam Hayter Williams Ramchandani Woodwards Dover Oldham Foster Stewart Smart Tate Newell Juniper Kendrick Ramsay-Baggs Patton Hall Brown Avery Awty Mellor Bailey Sadler Wood Bradley Barnard*

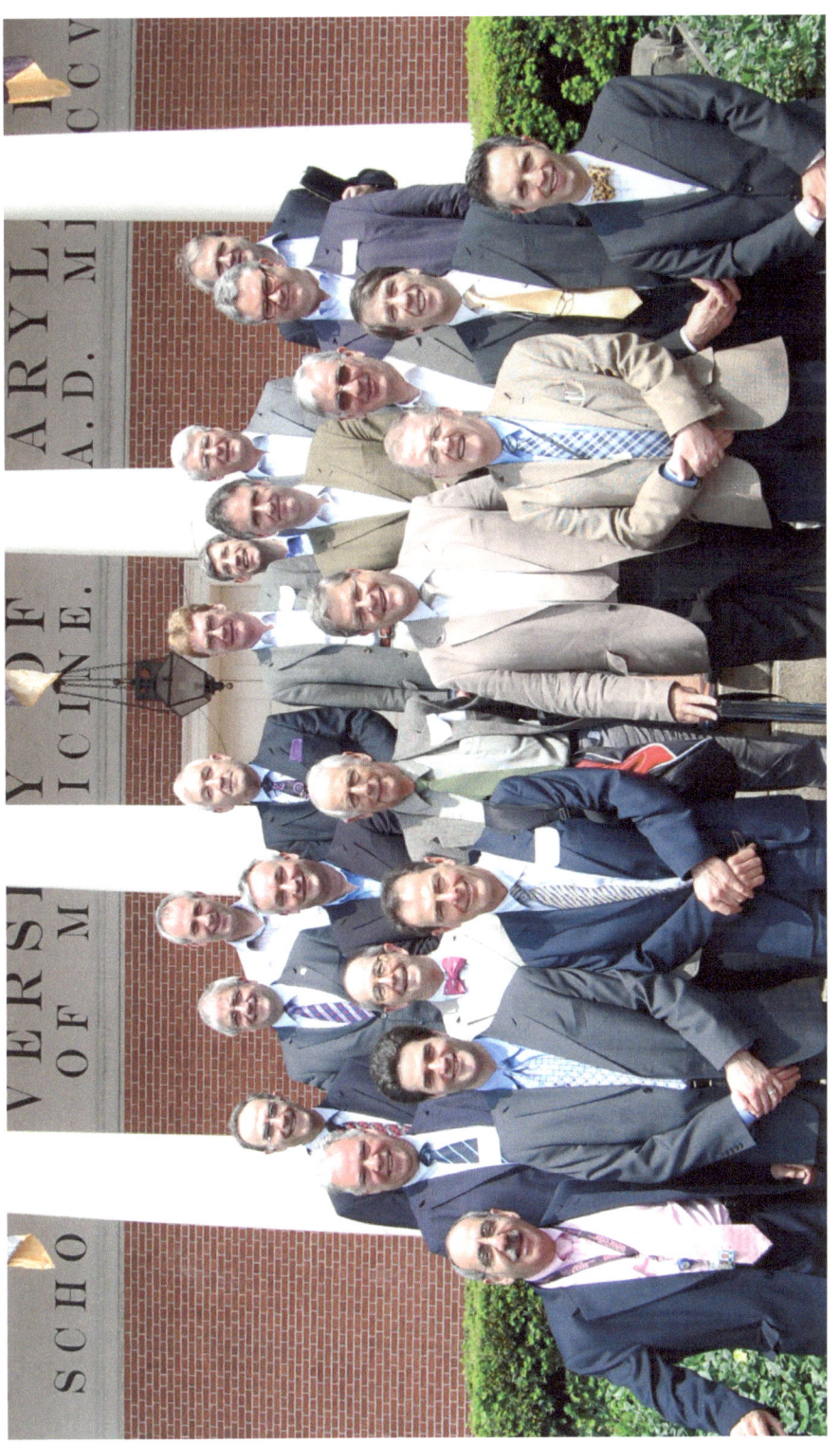

Baltimore May 2012

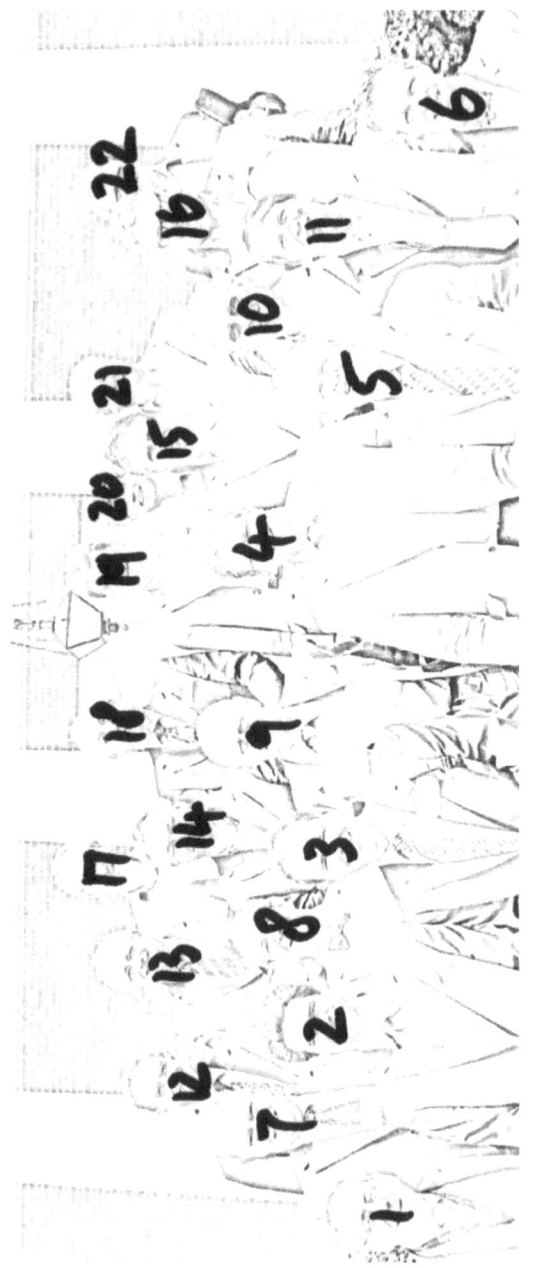

**Baltimore May 3-4 2012**
1 Dr Jaime Brahim, 2 Dr Joshua Lubek, 3 Lyons, 4 David Adlam President, 5 Bob Ord Host, 6 Dr John Caccamese, 7 Ramsay-Baggs, 8 Evans, 9 Oldham, 10 Avery, 11 Sadler, 12 Dr George Obeid, 13 Woodward, 14 Langton, 15 Martin, 16 Mellor, 17 Hislop, 18 Olley, 19 Boyd, 20 Koppel, 21 Lello, 22 Davidson

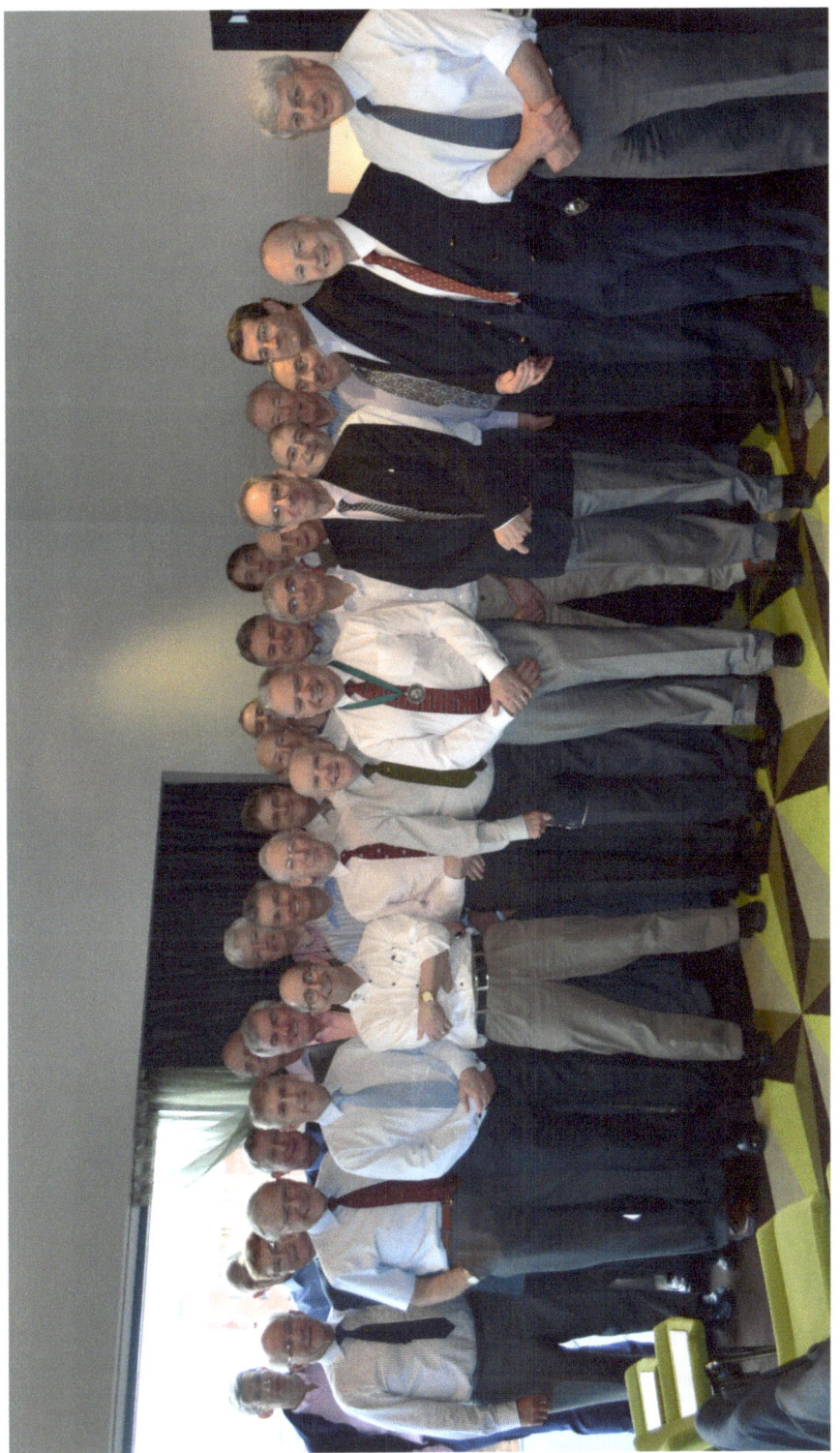

Belfast Nov 2013

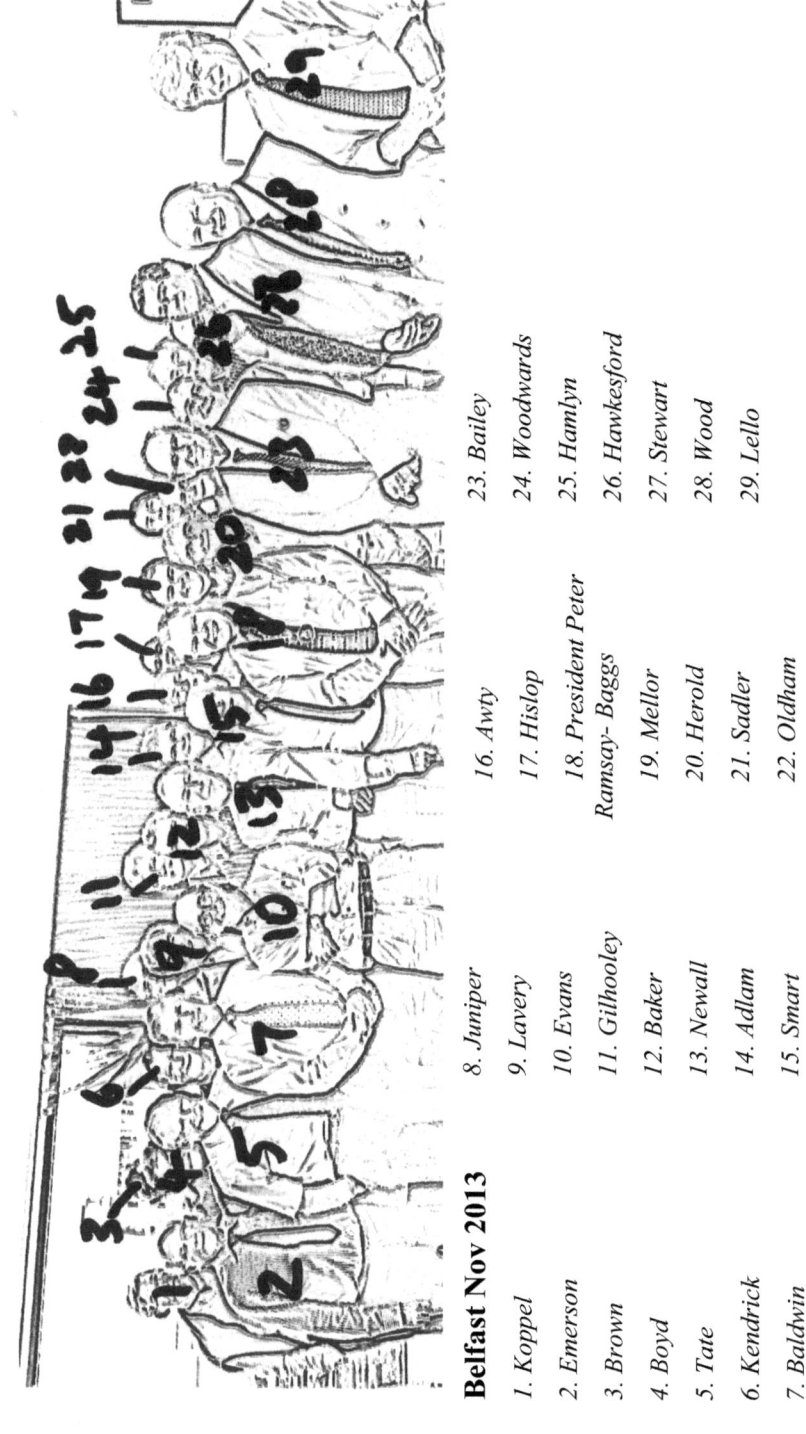

**Belfast Nov 2013**

1. Koppel
2. Emerson
3. Brown
4. Boyd
5. Tate
6. Kendrick
7. Baldwin
8. Juniper
9. Lavery
10. Evans
11. Gilhooley
12. Baker
13. Newall
14. Adlam
15. Smart
16. Awty
17. Hislop
18. President Peter Ramsay- Baggs
19. Mellor
20. Herold
21. Sadler
22. Oldham
23. Bailey
24. Woodwards
25. Hamlyn
26. Hawkesford
27. Stewart
28. Wood
29. Lello

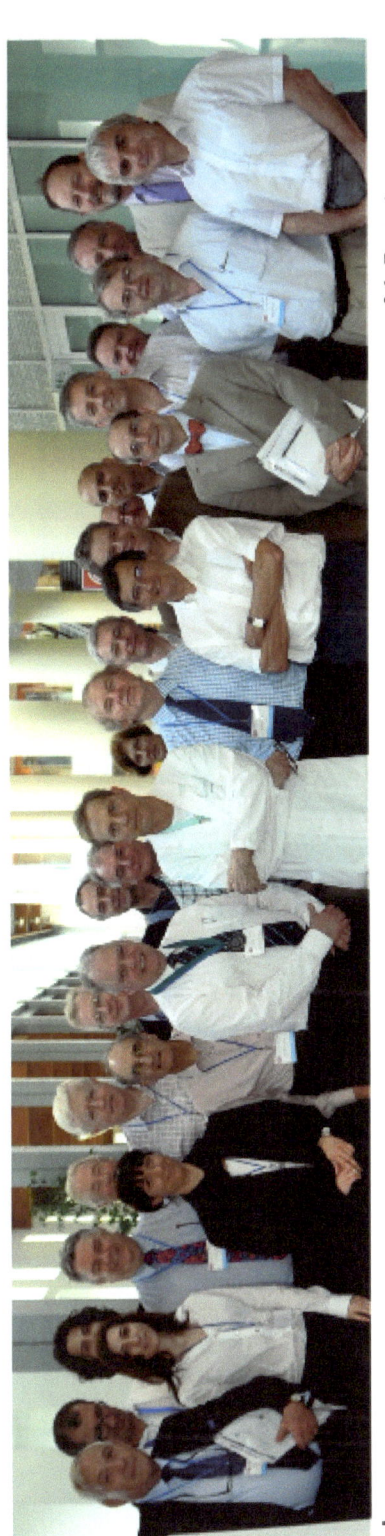

**Ferrara May 2013**

1. Olley
2. M Gaile
3. Unknown
4. Unknown
5. Mellor
6. Hamlyn
7. Unknown
8. Gilhooly
9. Moos
10. Hayter
11. President Peter Ramsey-Baggs
12. Hislop
13. Earl
14. Professor Clauser
15. Morton
16. Patton
17. Rowson
18. Ward Booth
19. Adlam
20. Penfold
21. Ramchandani
22. Evans
23. Cronin
24. McVicar
25. Davidson
26. Downie
27. Smith
28. Herold

79

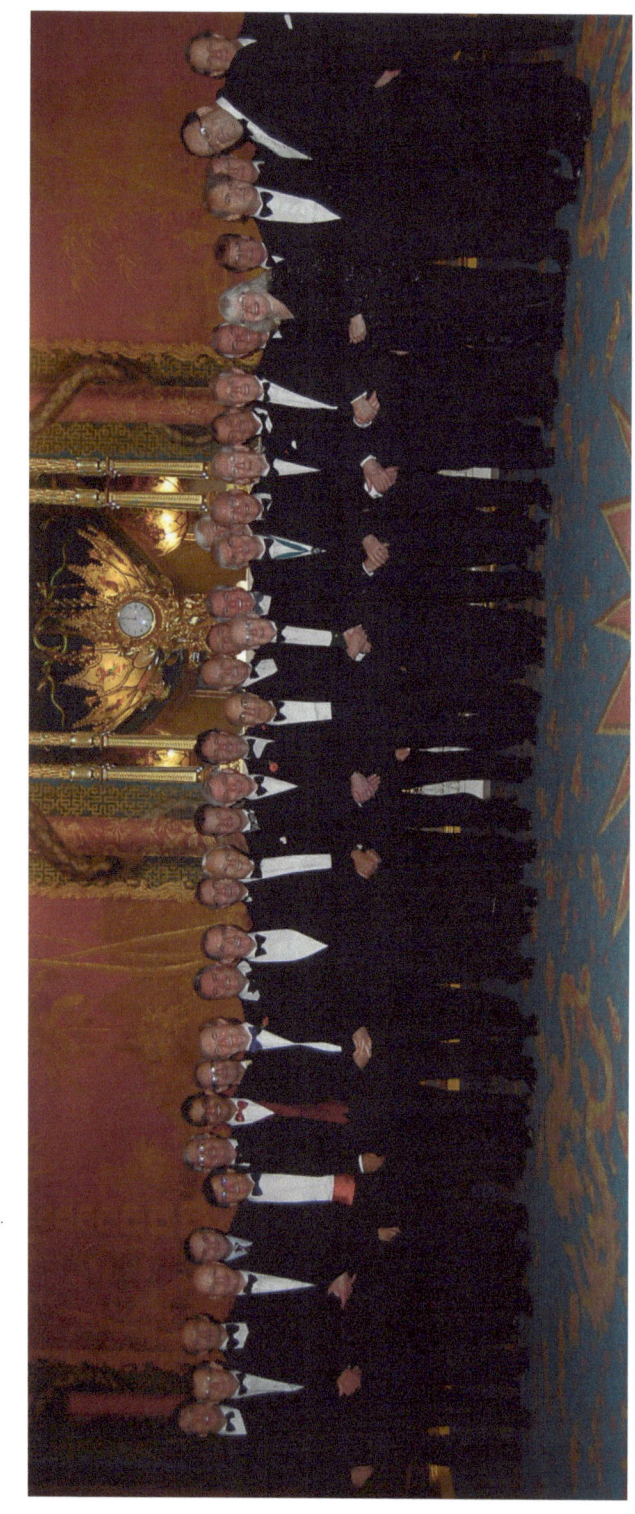

**Brighton Nov 7-9 2013**

**L-R**

*Sadler, Hall, Foster, Altman, Sneddon, Ward-Booth, Avery, Visavadia, Bailey, Patton, Mellor, Rowse, Hislop, Awty, Dover, Rowson, Martin, Moos, Brown, Revington, Smart, Lavery, President Jim Herold, Gilhooley, Tate, Newell, Camilleri, Baldwin, Earl, Fisher, Boyd, Davidson, Kendrick, Sugar, Simpson*

Prague April 2014

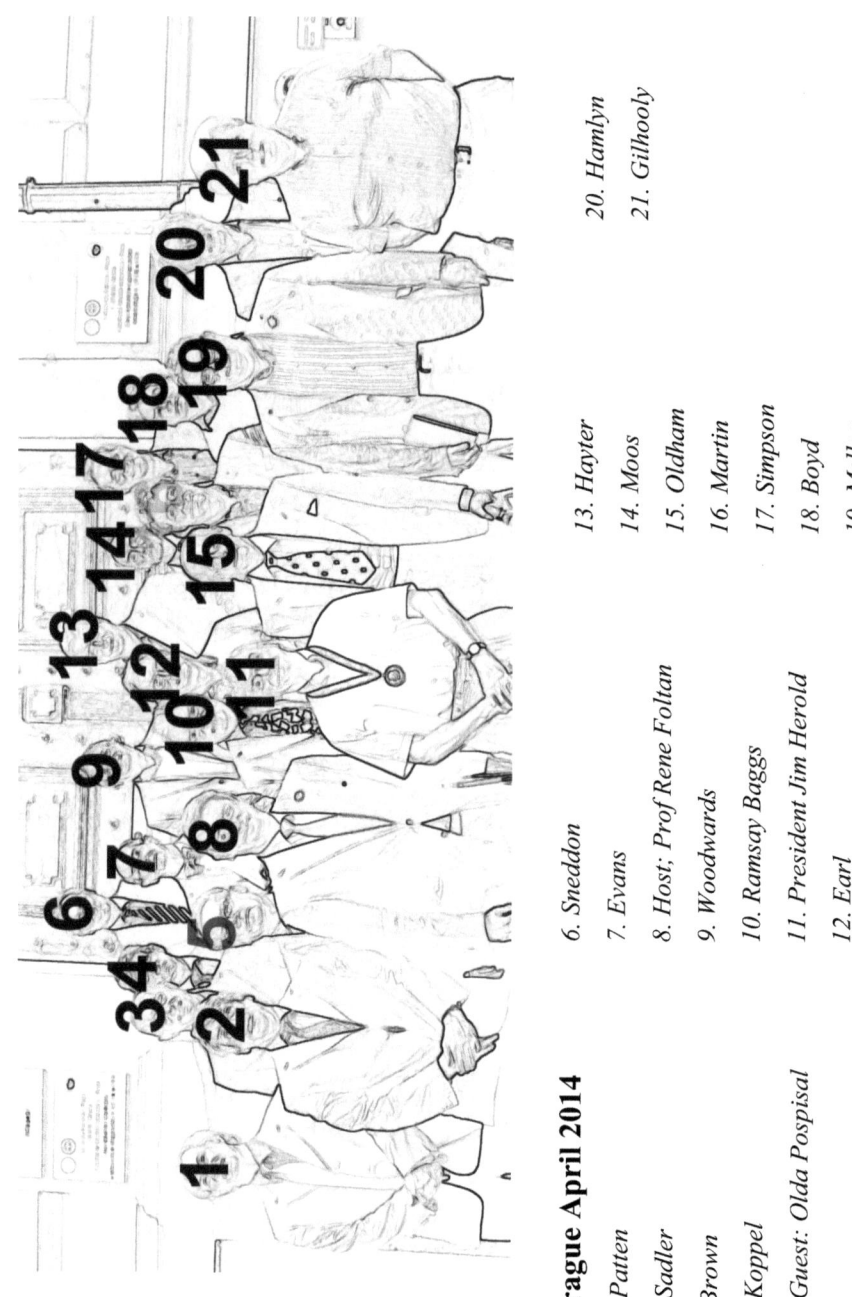

**Prague April 2014**

1. Patten
2. Sadler
3 Brown
4. Koppel
5. Guest: Olda Pospisal

6. Sneddon
7. Evans
8. Host; Prof Rene Foltan
9. Woodwards
10. Ramsay Baggs
11. President Jim Herold
12. Earl

13. Hayter
14. Moos
15. Oldham
16. Martin
17. Simpson
18. Boyd
19. Mellor

20. Hamlyn
21. Gilhooly

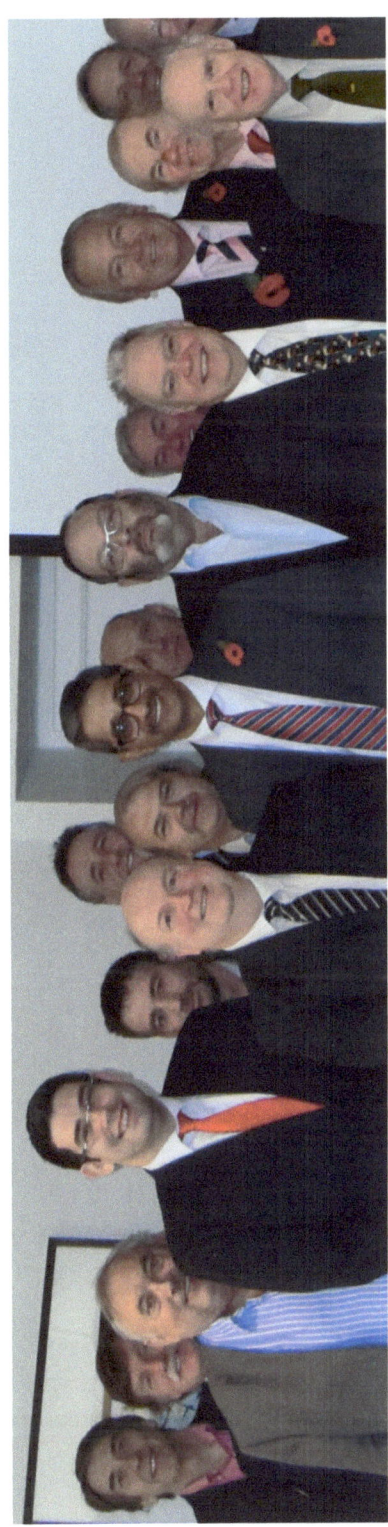

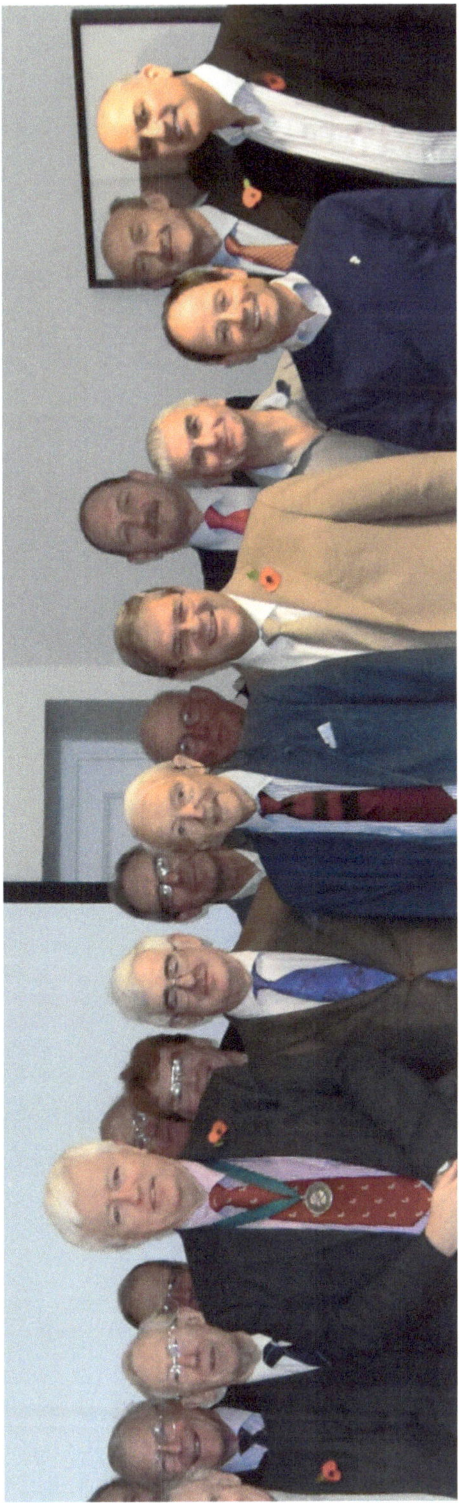

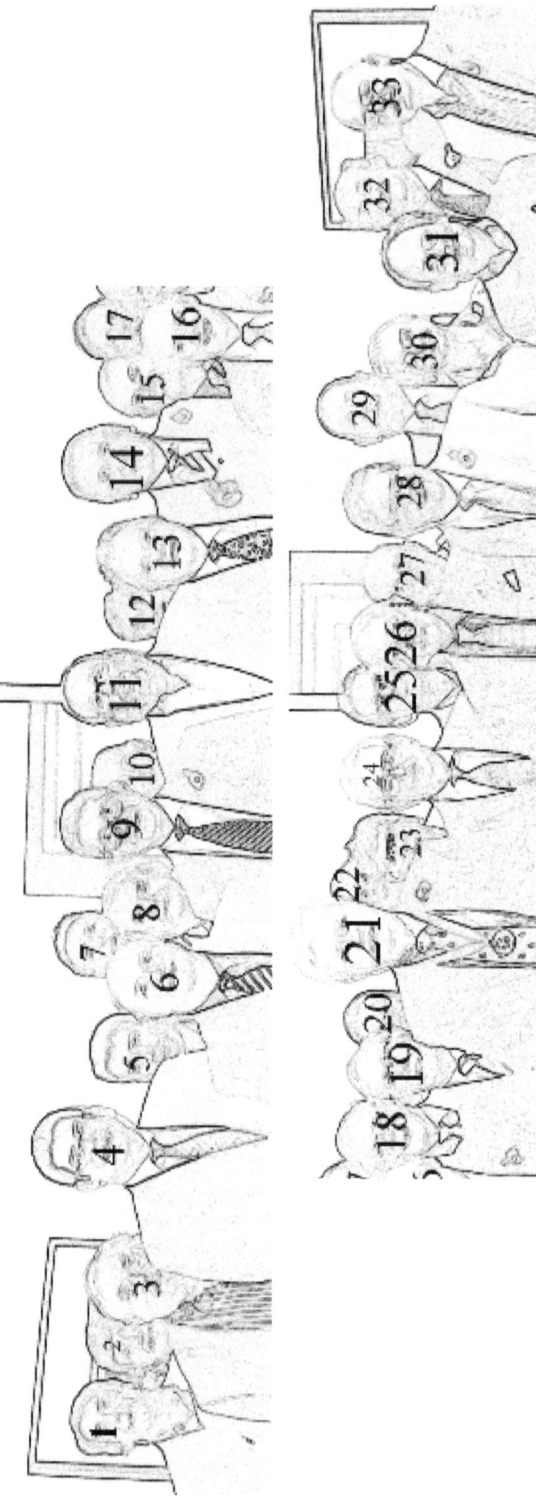

**Latimer Place 6–8th November 2014**

**Top L - R** 1. Sadler, 2. Renny 3. Hawkesford 4. Speaker Nick Sevdalis 5. Speaker Ross Doust 6. Speaker Mike Perry 7. Martin 8. Davidson 9. Visavadia 10. Brown 11. Sugar 12. Lavery 13. Ramsay-Baggs 14. Speaker Steve Cannon 15. Patten 16. Smart 17. Simpson **Bottom L - R** 18. Tate 19. Newell 20. Barnard 21. President Mick Gilhooly 22. Juniper 23. Boyd 24. Markus 25. Bailey 26. Awty 27. Banks 28. Adlam 29. Smith 30. Herold 31 Robinson 32 Foster 33. Ramchandani

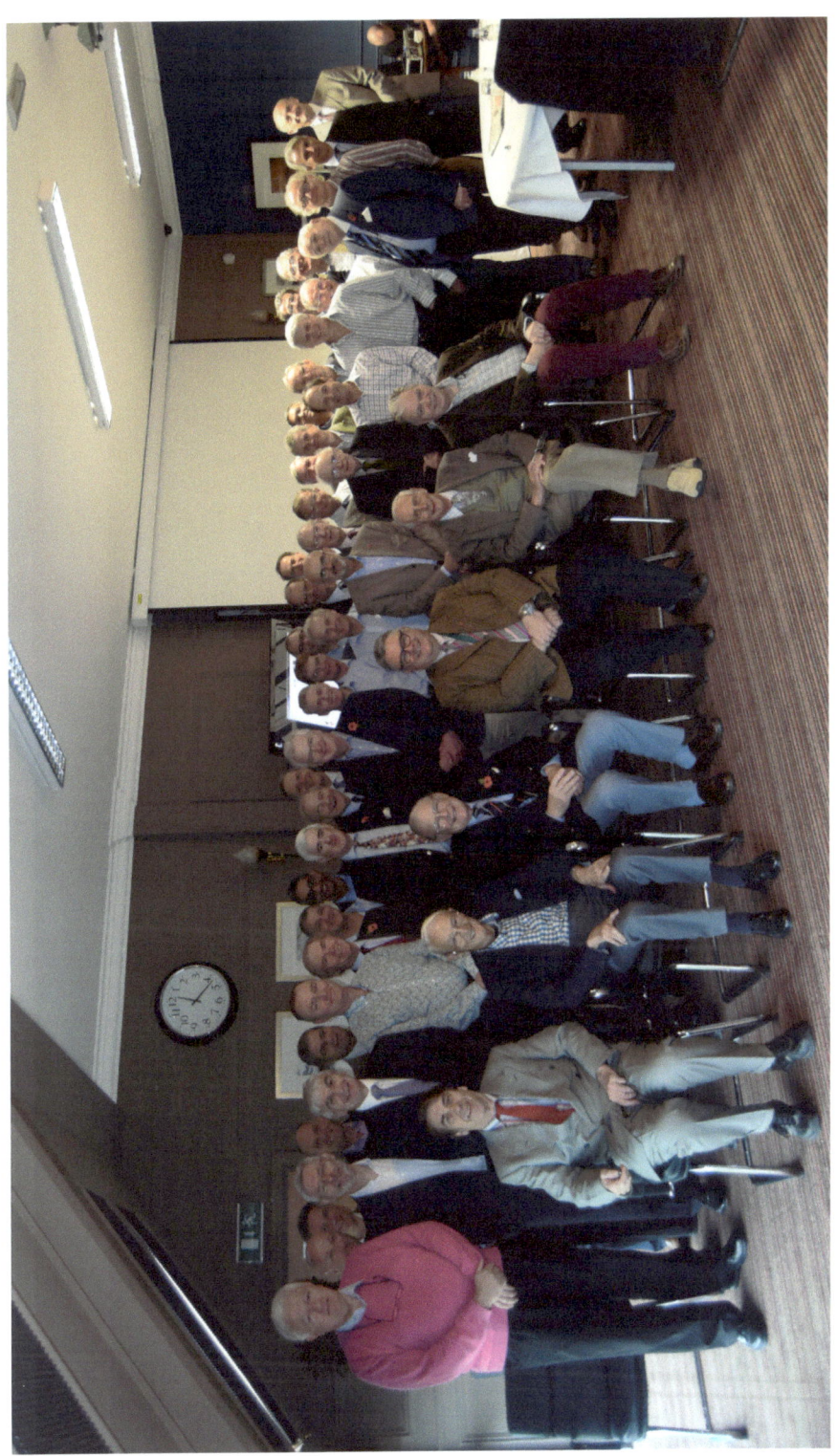

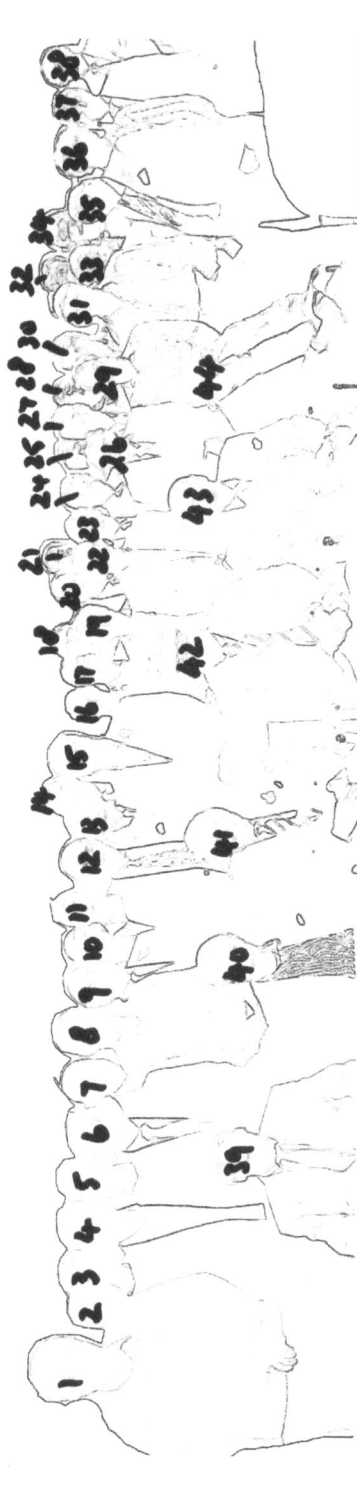

**Old Thorns 12th - 14th November 2015**

1. Gilhooly 2. Altman 3. Manolis 4. Rowson 5. Brown 6. Herold 7. Adlam 8. Revington 9. Patton 10. Camilleri 11. Visavadia 12.Markus 13. Williams 14. Simpson 15. Hayter16. Baldwin 17. Boyd 18. Hislop 19. Macpherson 20. Barnard 21. Lyons 22. Amin 23. Newall 24. Hall 25. Lavery 26. Smart 27. Baker 28. Kumar 29. Robinson 30. Bailey 31 Lello 32. Stewart 33. Earl 34. Avery 35. Olley 36. Patel 38. Foster 39. Sadler 40. Awty 41. Tate 42. President Tim Mellor 43. Oldham 44. Ramsay Baggs

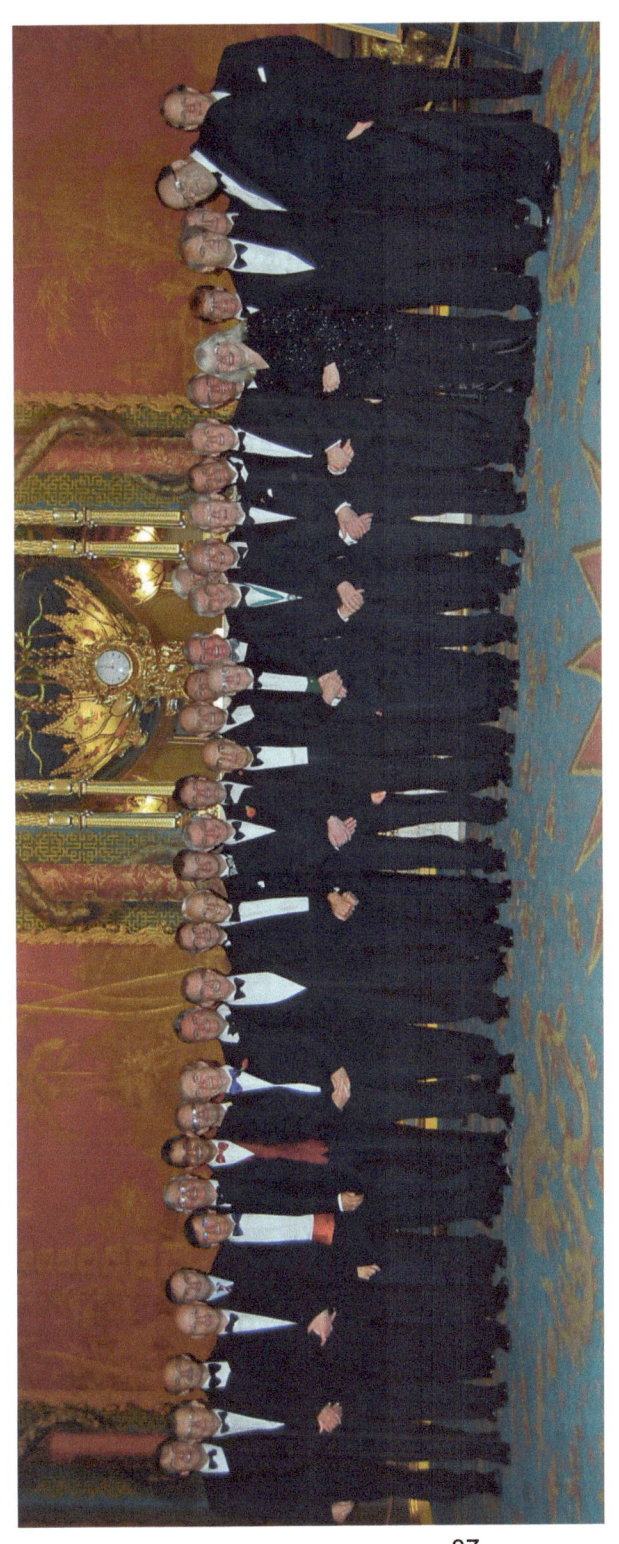

**Brighton November 9th 2014**

**Brighton November 9<sup>th</sup> 2014**

1. Sadler
2. Hall
3. Foster
4. Altman
5. Sneddon
6. Ward-Booth
7. Avery
8. Visavadia
9. Bailey
10. Patton
11. Mellor
12. Rowse
13. Hislop
14. Awty
15. Dover
16. Rowson
17. Martin
18. Moos
19. Brown
20. Revington
21. Smart
22. Lavery
23. President Jim Herold
24. Gilhooley
25. Tate
26. Newell
27. Camilleri
28. Baldwin
29. Earl
30. Fisher
31. Boyd
32. Davidson
33. Kendrick
34. Sugar
35. Simpson

88

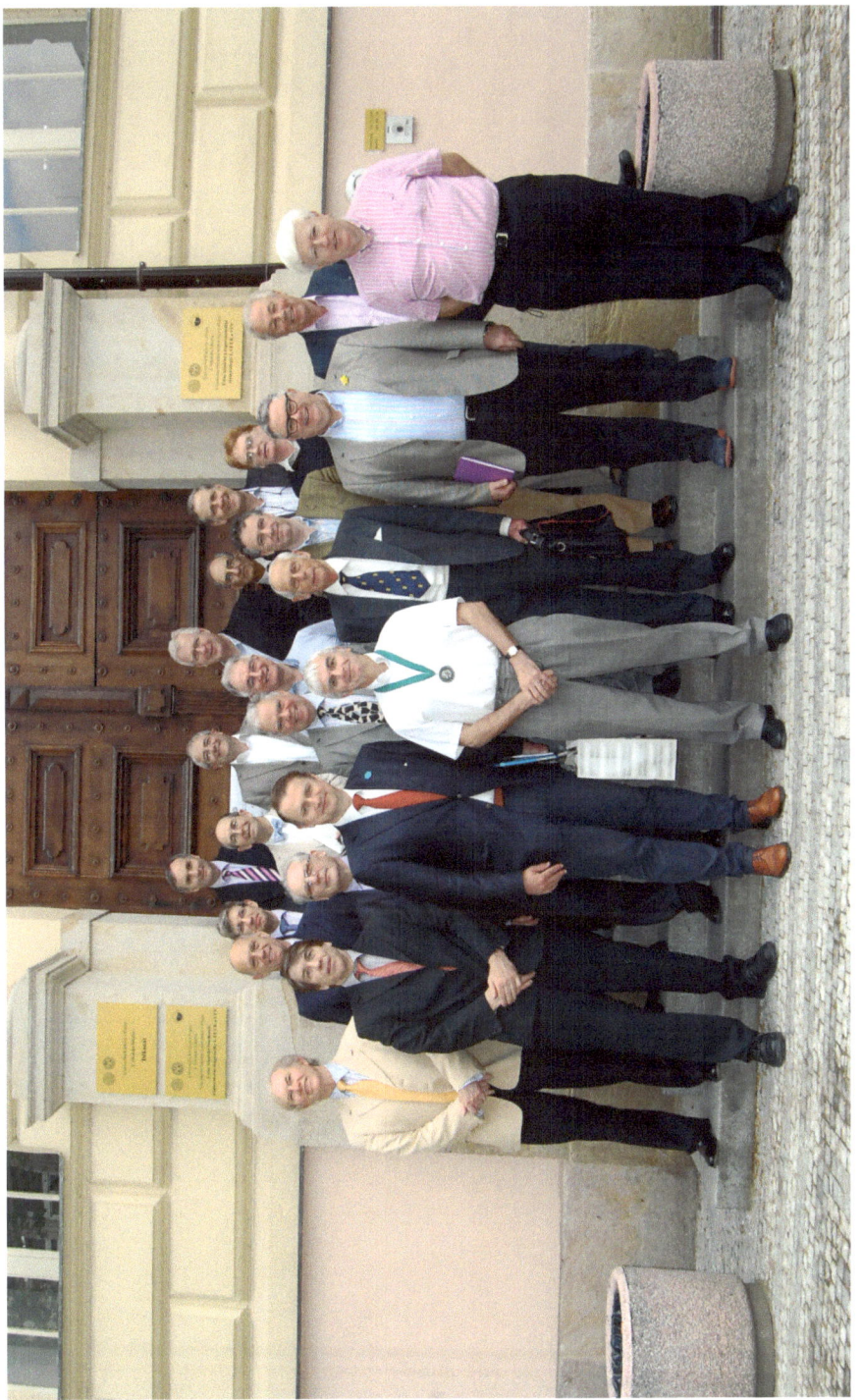

# Prague 25th April 2014

1. Patten
2. Sadler
3. Brown
4. Koppel
5. Guest: Olda Pospisal
6. Sneddon
7. Evans
8. Host; Prof Rene Foltan
9. Woodwards
10. Ramsay Baggs
11. President Jim Herold
12. Earl
13. Hayter
14. Moos
15. Oldham
16. Martin
17. Simpson
18. Boyd
19. Mellor
20. Hamlyn
21. Gillhooley

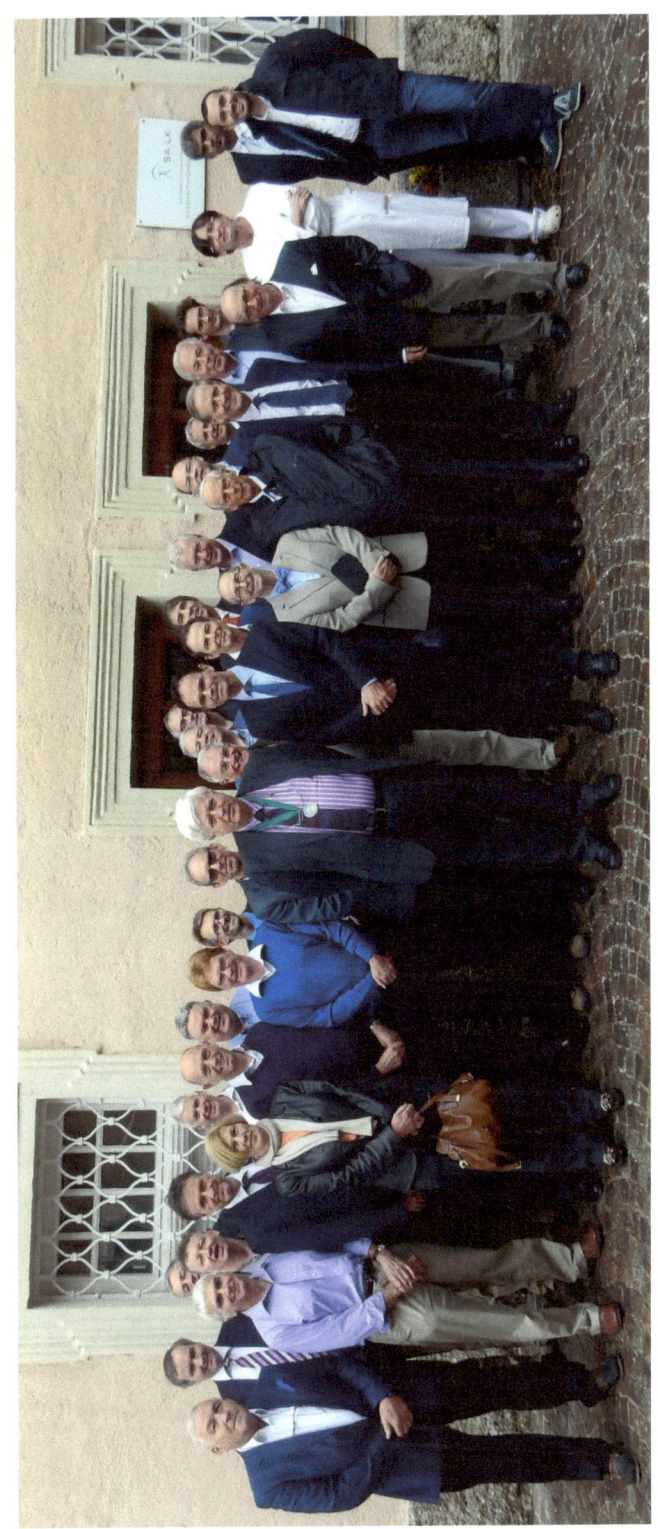

**Salzburg May 1st 2015**

OMF Surgeon, Salzburg 13. Malcolm Bailey
14. President Mick Gilbooley 15. Phil Earl
16. Peter Ramsay Baggs 17. Stuart Hislop
**Bottom L - R** 18. Host Professor A Gaggl
19. Andrew Lyons 20. Andrew Sadler 21.
Barry Evans 22. Jon Hayter 23. Laurence
Oldbam 24. Olaf Stanger Cardiac Surgeon
and our guide around hospital 25.Peter Sch-
achner OMF Surgeon, Salzburg 26. Mike
Simpson 27. John Hamlyn 28. Stephan
Granat Economic Director of hospital 29. ?
30. Johannes Hachleitner OMF Surgeon,
Salzburg 31 ? 32 Christoph Steiner OMF
Surgeon, Salzburg

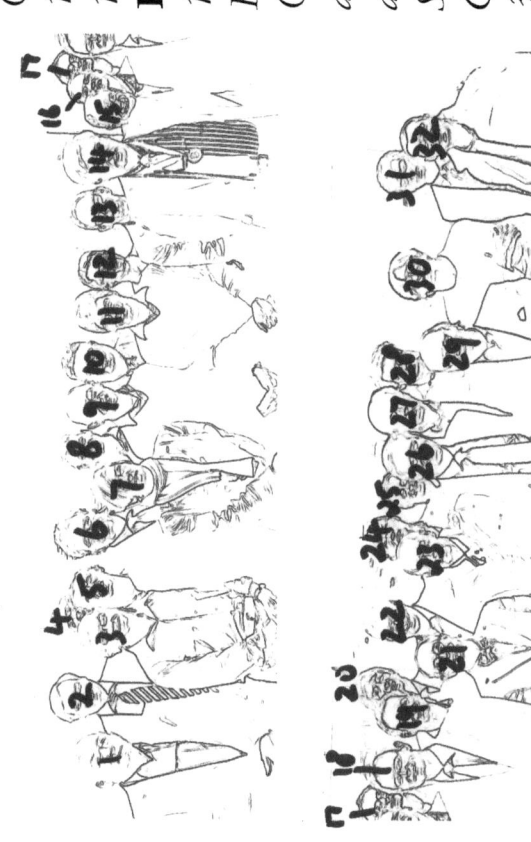

**Top L - R** 1. Steve Olley 2. Ken Sneddon 3. Jim
Herold 4. Carl Jones 5. Tony Patterson 6. Ian Martin
7. Maire Morton 8. Andrew Cronin 9. Andrew Brown
10. Tim Mellor 11. Bob Boyd 12.Christian Brandtner

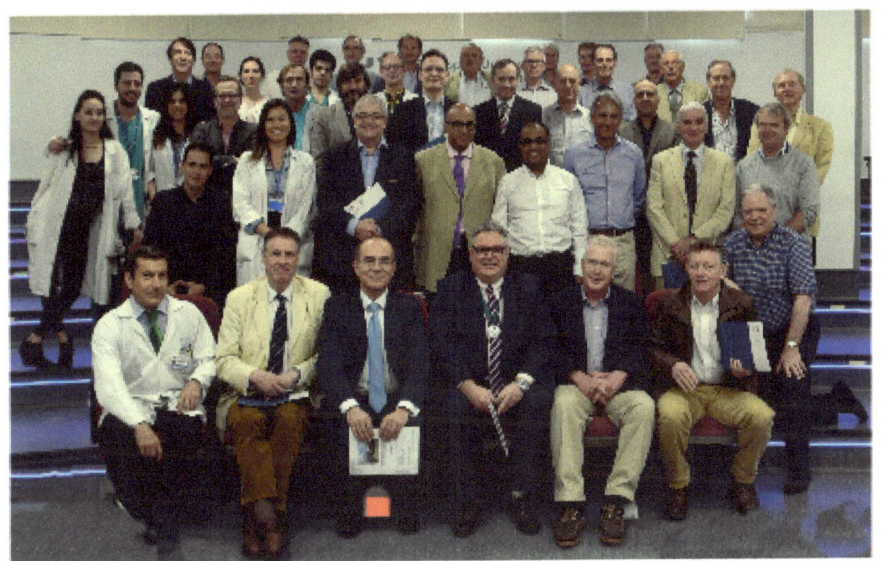

**Madrid May 2016**

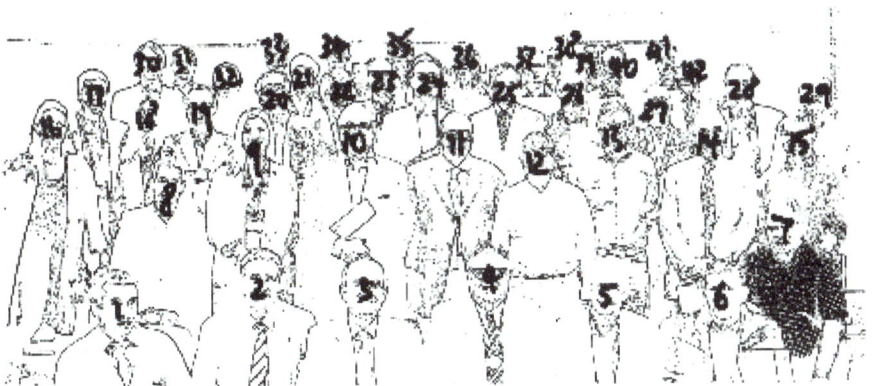

1. Dr M Picon
2. Martin
3. Host Professor Julio Acero
4. President Tim Mellor
5. Hayter
6. Patterson
7. Ramsay Baggs
8 ?
9. ?
10. Woodwards
11. Anand
12. Palmar
13. Patel
14. Herald

15. Davidson
16. ?
17. ?
18. ?
19. Dr F Almeida
20. Dr Jose Miguel Eslava Gurrea
21. ?
22. Dr E Sanchez Jauregui
23. ?
24. Norris
25. Sneddon
26. Brown
27. Katre

28. Simpson
29. Patton
30. Sadler
31. Robinson
32. ?
33. Heliotis
34. Hislop
35. Bentley
36. Hawkesford
37. Jones
38. Lello
39. Boyd
40. Lyons
41. Earl
42. Oldham

# Halifax May 2018

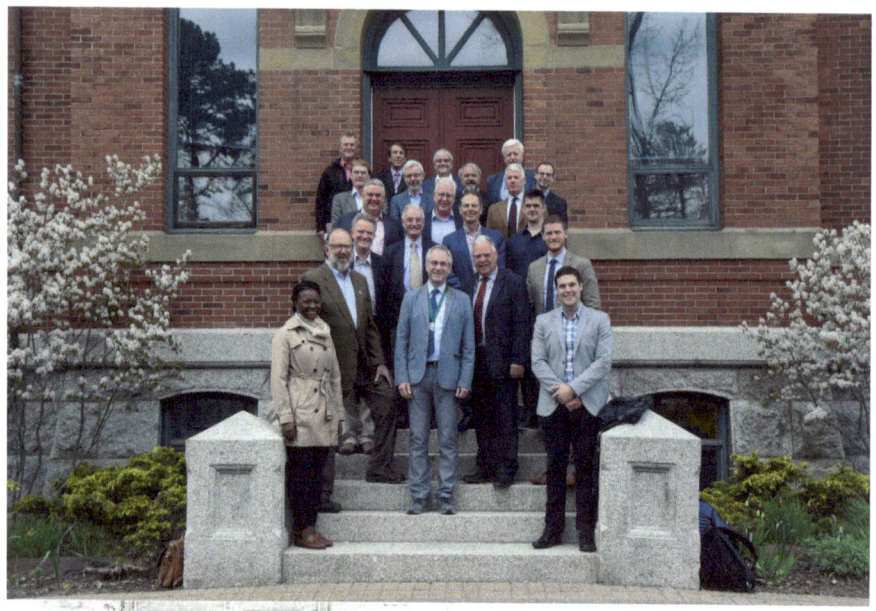

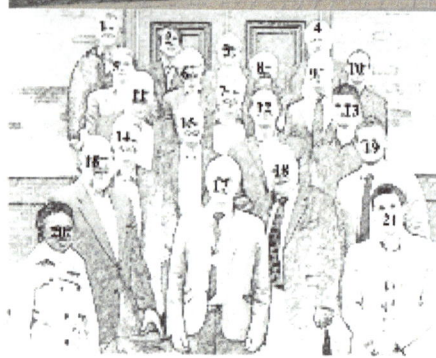

13. Dr Chad Robertson
14. McVicar
15. Earl
16. Dr Reginald Goodday
17. President Stuart Hislop
18. Ramsay Baggs
19. Dr Brad Fisher (Resident)
20. Dr Alero Boyo (Resident)
21. Dr Guy Barzan (Resident)

1. Dr Archie Morrison
2. Sadler
3. Woodwards
4. Gilhooly
5. Boyd
6. Rowson
7. Hayter
8. Davidson
9. Jones
10. Dr Jean-Charles Doucet
11. Mellor
12. Lyons

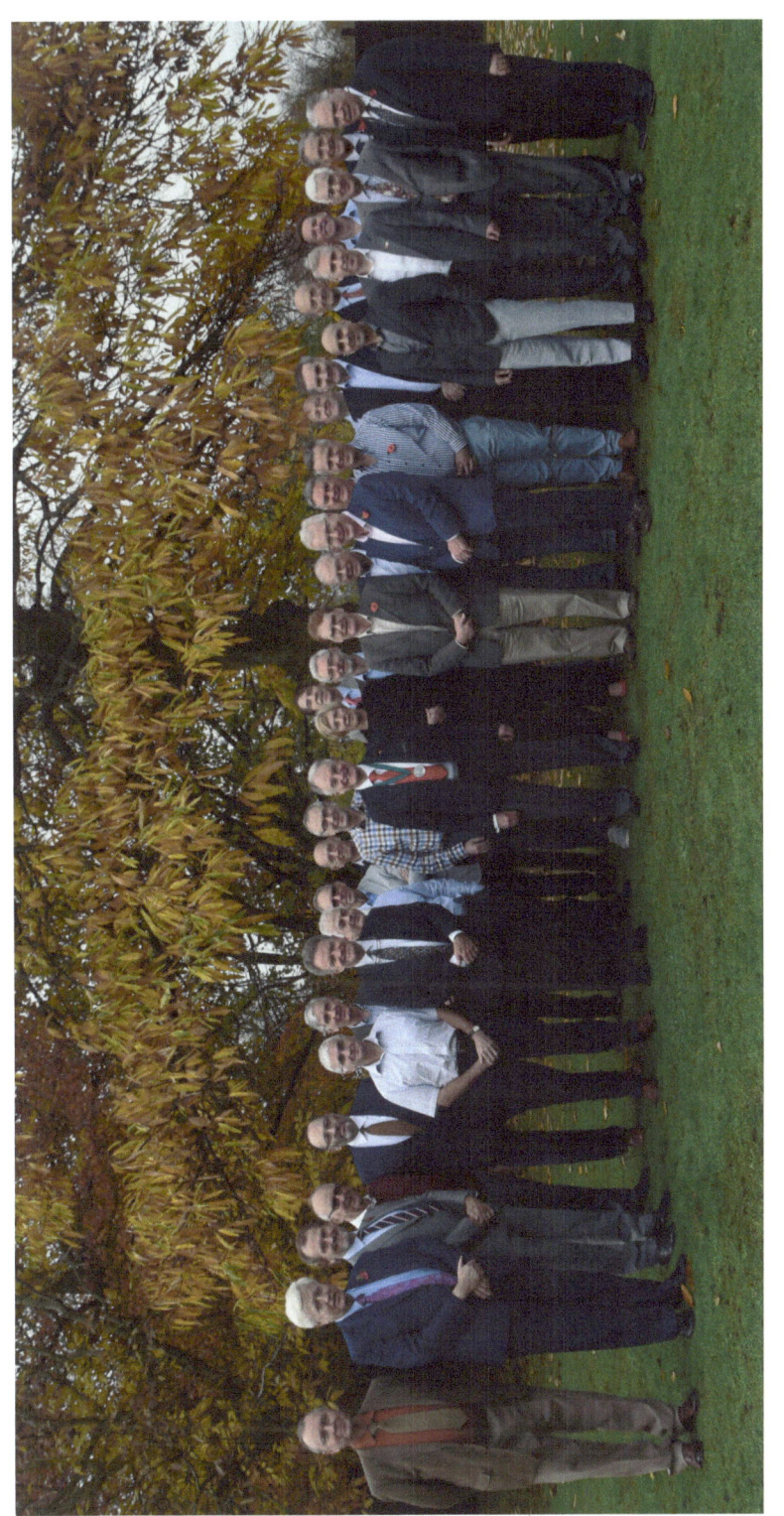

**Worcester November 2018**

# Lille May 2019

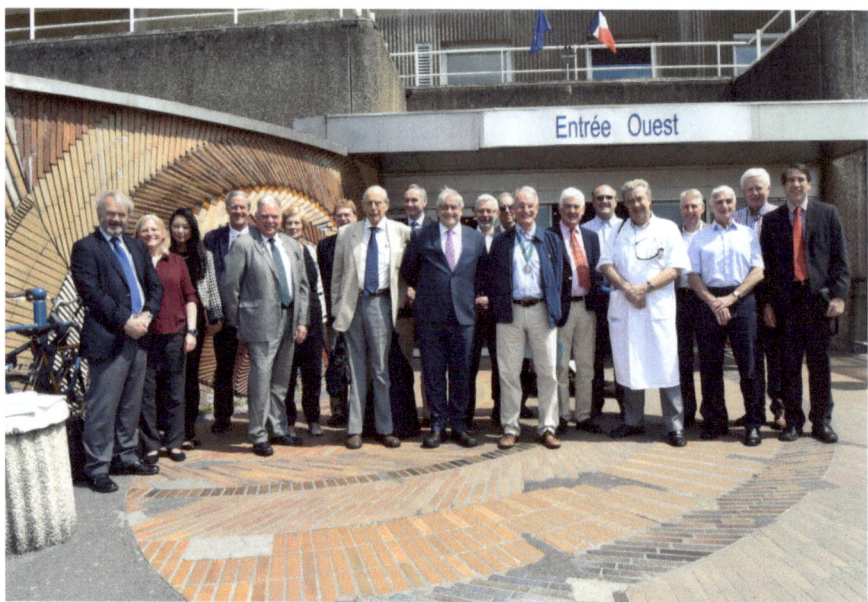

Left to right: Davidson, Beale, Fan, Simpson, Ramsay Baggs, Morton, Boyd, Oldham, Sneddon, Woodwards, Rowson, Bailey, Earl, Markus, Walsh, Host Professor Joël Ferri, Baldwin, Herold, Gilhooly, Sadler.

www.ingramcontent.com/pod-product-compliance
Lightning Source LLC
Chambersburg PA
CBHW040827180526
45159CB00001B/91